# RIBA Plan of Work 2013 Guide
# Health and Safety

CW01084146

**The RIBA Plan of Work 2013 Guides**

Other titles in the series:

*Design Management*, by Dale Sinclair

*Contract Administration*, by Ian Davies

*Information Exchanges*, by Richard Fairhead

*Project Leadership*, by Nick Willars

*Town Planning*, by Ruth Reed

*Sustainability*, by Sandy Halliday and Richard Atkins

Coming soon:

*Conservation*, by Hugh Feilden

The RIBA Plan of Work 2013 is endorsed by the following organisations:

Royal Incorporation of
Architects in Scotland

Chartered Institute of
Architectural Technologists

Royal Society of
Architects in Wales

Construction
Industry Council

Royal Society
of Ulster Architects

RIBA Plan of Work 2013 Guide

# Health and Safety

**Peter Caplehorn**

RIBA Publishing

© RIBA Enterprises Ltd, 2016
Published by RIBA Publishing, The Old Post Office, St Nicholas Street,
Newcastle upon Tyne NF1 1RH

ISBN 978 1 85946 588 2
Stock code 83976

British Library Cataloguing in Publication Data
A catalogue record for this book is available from the British Library.

Commissioning Editor: Sarah Busby
Series Editor: Dale Sinclair
Project Manager: Alasdair Deas
Design: Kneath Associates
Typesetting: Academic+Technical, Bristol, UK
Printed and bound by CPI Group (UK) Ltd
Cover image: © Christian Richters/VIEW

Picture credits
Figure 2.2 is reproduced from HSE publication L153, under the terms
of the Open Government Licence.

RIBA Publishing is part of RIBA Enterprises Ltd
www.ribaenterprises.com

# Contents

# Foreword

CDM 2015 provides a flexible regulatory framework through which clients, supported by their principal designers and principal contractors, can determine the most effective arrangements for designing and delivering every construction project in a safe and healthy manner.

Although new to CDM 2015, the role of principal designer now brings to risk management and planning in the preconstruction phase what the principal contractor has successfully provided in the construction phase for many years.

The benefits to design risk management and subsequent risk reduction in the construction phase will be increasingly realised as the industry moves ever closer toward appointing and embedding the principal designer role from the outset and at the heart of every preconstruction phase.

HSE acknowledges and welcomes all industry initiatives and publications, such as this guide written by Peter Caplehorn, where they help dutyholders understand and meet their obligations under the Regulations in a sensible and proportionate way – thereby delivering a safer and healthier construction industry in the 21st century.

**Simon Longbottom**
*Head of Construction Sector*
*Health and Safety Executive*

# Series editor's foreword

The RIBA Plan of Work 2013 was developed in response to the needs of an industry adjusting to emerging digital design processes, disruptive technologies and new procurement models, as well as other drivers. A core challenge is to communicate the thinking behind the new RIBA Plan in greater detail. This process is made more complex because the RIBA Plan of Work has existed for 50 years and is embodied within the psyche and working practices of everyone involved in the built environment sector. Its simplicity has allowed it to be interpreted and used in many ways, underpinning the need to explain the content of the Plan's first significant edit. By relating the Plan to a number of commonly encountered topics, the *RIBA Plan of Work 2013 Guides* series forms a core element of the communication strategy and I am delighted to be acting as the series editor.

The first strategic shift in the RIBA Plan of Work 2013 was to acknowledge a change from the tasks of the design team to those of the project team: the client, design team and contractor. Stages 0 and 7 are part of this shift, acknowledging that buildings are used by clients, or their clients, and, more importantly, recognising the paradigm shift from designing for construction towards the use of high-quality design information to help facilitate better whole-life outcomes.

New procurement strategies focused around assembling the right project team are the beginnings of significant adjustments in the way that buildings will be briefed, designed, constructed, operated and used. Design teams are harnessing new digital design technologies (commonly bundled under the BIM wrapper), linking geometric information to new engineering analysis software to create a generation of buildings that would not previously have been possible. At the same time, coordination processes and environmental credentials are being improved. A core focus is the progressive fixity of high-quality information – for the first time, the right information at the right time, clearly defining who does what, when.

The RIBA Plan of Work 2013 aims to raise the knowledge bar on many subjects, including sustainability, Information Exchanges and health and safety. The *RIBA Plan of Work 2013 Guides* are crucial tools in disseminating and explaining how these themes are fully addressed and how the new Plan can be harnessed to achieve the new goals and objectives of our clients.

**Dale Sinclair**
*April 2016*

# Acknowledgements and dedication

I would like to acknowledge the help and support of Paul Bussey, Adrian Dobson, Jane Duncan, Richard Brindley and Andrew Townsend (in memoriam), my many colleagues at the Health and Safety Executive, including Philip White, Peter Barker, Simon Longbottom and Russell Addfield, the CIC Health and Safety Committee, colleagues at RIBA Publishing, and the RIBA Regulations and Standards Group.

I would also like to thank my partner, Pearl, for her support and encouragement.

This book is dedicated to the many people whose lives, every year, are seriously affected by their involvement with the construction industry.

# About the author

Peter Caplehorn RIBA HonMCIAT is a chartered architect with more than 35 years' experience in the construction industry. For more than 15 years he has engaged with the wider industry in a number of key national roles and has represented the industry in many media positions.

For 14 years Peter was Technical Director at the architectural practice Scott Brownrigg, but in 2014 he took up the role of Deputy Chief Executive at the Construction Products Association. Peter's role includes the development of many current themes across the industry, including better, smarter regulations and standards, innovation, Building Information Modelling (BIM), sustainable construction and energy efficiency.

He has expert knowledge of UK construction regulations and health and safety and is currently working closely with the RIBA, British Standards Institution, BRE, Department for Business, Innovation and Skills and the Health and Safety Executive. He has been central to the delivery of several British Standards and Publicly Available Specifications.

Peter was a RIBA Council Member from 2009 to 2014 and a founder member of the Designers' Initiative on Health and Safety (DIOHAS). In 2015 he was awarded honorary membership of CIAT, and he has been a CIBSE associate member since 2010. His current industry roles include:

I  RIBA Health and Safety Champion
I  CIC Executive Board member and Health and Safety Champion
I  Building Regulations Advisory Committee deputy chair
I  BSI: Standards Policy and Strategy Committee member and chair of the Construction and Built Environment Committee
I  BRE Standing Panel member
I  BIM4Regs chair.

Currently, he is involved with the use of BIM and health and safety, is a member of the Health in Construction leadership group and is working with the Bonfield Review on energy efficiency.

# About the series editor

Dale Sinclair is Director of Technical Practice for AECOM's architecture team in EMIA.

His core expertise is the delivery of large-scale projects and he is passionate about delivering these more effectively using innovative and iterative multidisciplinary design processes that embrace the project life cycle, manage the iterative design process and improve design outcomes. He believes that the lead designer's role is central to this goal and his publication *Leading the Team: An Architect's Guide to Design Management* is aimed at those who share these objectives.

He regularly lectures on BIM, design management, the future of the built environment industry and the RIBA Plan of Work 2013.

He is currently the RIBA President's Ambassador for Industry Collaboration and Technical Innovation, the CIC BIM Champion and a UK board member of BuildingSMART. He authored the *BIM Overlay to the Outline Plan of Work 2007*, edited the RIBA Plan of Work 2013 and was author of its supporting tools and guidance publications: *Guide to Using the RIBA Plan of Work 2013* and *Assembling a Collaborative Project Team*.

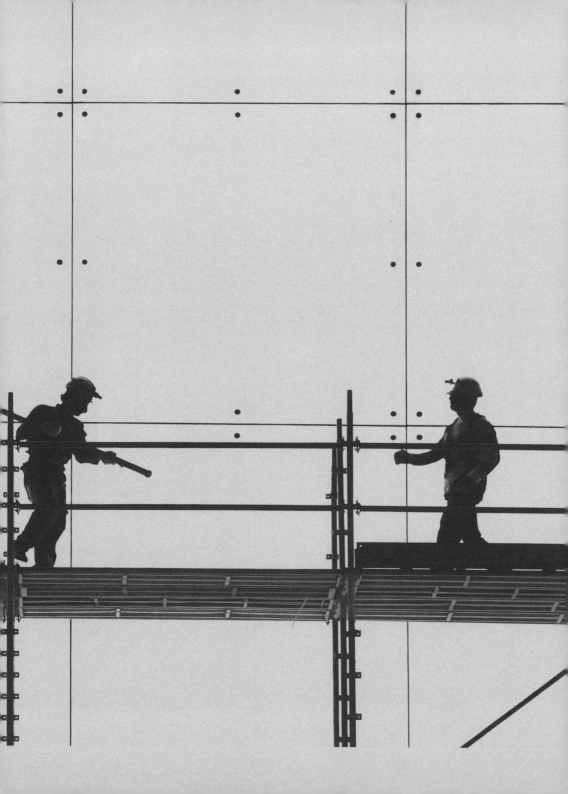

# Introduction

## Health and safety

Health and safety is a core part of any business operation. It is not an 'add on', nor is it something to be looked at with disdain or misplaced humour. It is essential that every construction project team member has an understanding of the subject – it is as important as an appreciation of good design, good interpersonal skills and proficiency in business planning.

Construction is still one of the most unsafe sectors in which to work. While progress has been made, on average one person is killed and several dozen are injured every week in the UK in construction-related accidents. Everyone in the industry has a responsibility to help consign these statistics to history.

Many workers are also subjected to long-term health hazards. Manual handling and exposure to dust particulates, solar radiation and volatile organic compounds (VOCs) can all generate health problems that might not emerge until decades later. There is a tendency to overlook these long-term health issues – the aim must be to treat health like safety.

## The business risk

In the modern world an inability to grasp a core subject is a severe business risk. Therefore, every designer needs to attain a grounded competence in health and safety and understand its relevance to day-to-day practice.

That is not to say that everyone should become a health and safety zealot. Rather, having an understanding of this area is important as it builds confidence: confidence in advising clients, confidence in running projects and confidence in business planning. This should lead to health and safety principles being applied across projects in a sensible and well-rounded manner.

## Health and safety and the RIBA Plan of Work 2013

Health and safety considerations have been embedded in the RIBA Plan of Work 2013 from the outset, recognising the importance of the subject. Indeed, health and safety is an essential consideration throughout any project; from the framing of the strategy, through the development of the design and the planning of construction work on site, to the actual use of the building.

A Health and Safety Strategy must be established for every project – it will be the constant thread that runs through the project. The importance of this strategy cannot be overstated.

Stage outputs are identified in the RIBA Plan of Work 2013. It is essential that these are used as milestones, to ensure that a project is on track and progressing well. They are also a requirement for any government work.

Statutory regulation – and health and safety regulation in particular – is ever present through this framework. However, while complying with regulations will ensure that any operations meet the legal requirements, good practice should always go beyond the minimum required standards – raising the bar as high as possible. *so not stairs*

## Regulation is an important starting point

It is essential to have a correct understanding of any relevant regulations, otherwise the statutory requirements and responsibilities contained in those regulations may not be fully appreciated. This applies across all spheres of regulation, not just health and safety.

Regulations are often misquoted, abbreviated or reported entirely out of context. Health and safety regulations, in particular, seem to attract misinterpretation, which serves only to muddy the waters for anyone attempting to understand their obligations and how to comply with them. It should also be remembered that all regulations have context and a 'sphere of influence', so it is vital to understand how they fit into the wider picture.

Much of UK construction regulation is based around target setting principles, rather than prescriptive requirements. While this is deliberate – to enable innovation in the industry – it increases the risk of misinterpretation and debate.

Many regulations are applied by custom and practice, commonly described as 'deemed to satisfy' or even 'rule of thumb'. Convention is often confused with regulation, which can give rise to arguments and procedural conflict.

## Begin with good practice

Start as you mean to go on. While this may seem obvious advice, it is critical for the initial stages of any project. This is when the character of everything going forward is established. Have in mind the types of actions likely to be required in the stages to come, the nature of your role in the project and the input the client is expecting you to provide.

For there to be any chance of delivering the client's Project Objectives, clarity, organisation and understanding are needed. Many design team members setting out on a new project will focus their energy on the client and on the development of the Initial Project Brief. Designers in particular are driven by the thought of original creation. This is what fuels enthusiasm and energy, but it needs to be balanced with the application of logic and experience.

After the initial enthusiasm – creation of the initial concept – there must be a consideration of how this can be achieved. This is when the health and safety thread (among many others) must start to be drawn. It must be included from the start, and must continue to be carried through the rest of the project, right through to completion and handover.

Health and safety seems to be one of those issues that attracts either too much or too little attention. It is often treated either in an overly keen and bureaucratic way – often resulting in the easy goals being missed – or is simply paid lip service, in an 'it's not for us' style. Obviously, neither of these approaches is correct. We should always be attempting to apply the 'Goldilocks' principle – not too little and not too much. The Health and Safety Strategy must consider the regulations, when needed, address the project principles, when needed, and ensure that the client's team and the contractor are fully connected, when needed.

## Health and safety and the RIBA Plan of Work 2013

Health and safety needs to be considered throughout all the stages of the RIBA Plan of Work 2013, running the whole length of the project. It will, of course, become more relevant in some stages than in others – a point that is often missed by those outside the design community. Design is intrinsically an iterative process and so will develop through the project; therefore, there must be space to allow it to develop successfully. Having a health and safety straightjacket imposed the whole time is not viable.

While the design is being developed, health and safety considerations – while present in the background – should be relaxed so that they do not stifle creative design. However, they must be brought to the fore when tangible design progress has been made. This proportionate approach needs an appropriate organisational structure.

The RIBA Plan of Work 2013 has been structured around a coordinated approach across the construction industry. One aspect required for UK Government work is a series of Information Exchanges. These are particularly important when projects use a Building Information Modelling (BIM) methodology. Information Exchanges may be required at every stage.

Getting prepared is also about learning from the past. The RIBA Plan of Work 2013 makes learning from previous projects – from Stage 7 information – an essential part of developing expertise for the future. Lessons learned from previous projects should be fed into developing new processes and structures for the next. Cleaning and maintenance organisation, information sharing across the team, new software or meetings – all can be made more effective.

Do it well this time, with the right approach, and it can be even better next time.

Peter Caplehorn
*April 2016*

## Using this series

For ease of reference each book in this series is broken down into chapters that map on to the stages of the Plan of Work. So, for instance, the first chapter covers the tasks and considerations around health and safety at Stage 0.

We have also included several in-text features to enhance your understanding of the topic. The following key will explain what each icon means and why each feature is useful to you:

 The 'Example' feature explores an example from practice, either real or theoretical

 The 'Tools and Templates' feature outlines standard tools, letters and forms and how to use them in practice

 The 'Signpost' feature introduces you to further sources of trusted information from books, websites and regulations

 The 'Definition' feature explains key terms in this topic area in more detail

 The 'Hints and Tips' feature dispenses pragmatic advice and highlights common problems and solutions

 The 'Small Project Observation' feature highlights useful variations in approach and outcome for smaller projects

# RIBA

The **RIBA Plan of Work 2013** organises the process of briefing, designing, constructing, maintaining, operating and using building projects into a number of key stages. The content of stages may vary or overlap to suit specific project requirements.

**RIBA Plan of Work 2013**

**Stages**

**Tasks ▼**

| | 0 Strategic Definition | 1 Preparation and Brief | 2 Concept Design | 3 Developed Design |
|---|---|---|---|---|
| Core Objectives | Identify client's **Business Case** and **Strategic Brief** and other core project requirements. | Develop **Project Objectives**, including **Quality Objectives** and **Project Outcomes**, **Sustainability Aspirations**, **Project Budget**, other parameters or constraints and develop **Initial Project Brief**. Undertake **Feasibility Studies** and review of **Site Information**. | Prepare **Concept Design**, including outline proposals for structural design, building services systems, outline specifications and preliminary **Cost Information** along with relevant **Project Strategies** in accordance with **Design Programme**. Agree alterations to brief and issue **Final Project Brief**. | Prepare **Developed Design**, including coordinated and updated proposals for structural design, building services systems, outline specifications, **Cost Information** and **Project Strategies** in accordance with **Design Programme**. |
| Procurement *Variable task bar | Initial considerations for assembling the project team. | Prepare **Project Roles Table** and **Contractual Tree** and continue assembling the project team. | ⊰⁻ The procurement strategy does not fundamentally alter the progression of the design or the level of detail prepared at | a given stage. However, **Information Exchanges** will vary depending on the selected procurement route and **Building Contract**. A bespoke **RIBA Plan of Work** |
| Programme *Variable task bar | Establish **Project Programme**. | Review **Project Programme**. | Review **Project Programme**. | ⊰⁻ The procurement route may dictate the **Project Programme** and result in certain stages overlapping |
| (Town) Planning *Variable task bar | Pre-application discussions. | Pre-application discussions. | ⊰⁻ Planning applications are typically made using the Stage 3 output. | A bespoke **RIBA Plan of Work 2013** will identify when the |
| Suggested Key Support Tasks | Review **Feedback** from previous projects. | Prepare **Handover Strategy** and **Risk Assessments**. Agree **Schedule of Services**, **Design Responsibility Matrix** and **Information Exchanges** and prepare **Project Execution Plan** including **Technology** and **Communication Strategies** and consideration of **Common Standards** to be used. | Prepare **Sustainability Strategy, Maintenance and Operational Strategy** and review **Handover Strategy** and **Risk Assessments**. Undertake third party consultations as required and any **Research and Development** aspects. Review and update **Project Execution Plan**. Consider **Construction Strategy**, including offsite fabrication, and develop **Health and Safety Strategy**. | Review and update **Sustainability, Maintenance and Operational** and **Handover Strategies** and **Risk Assessments**. Undertake third party consultations as required and conclude **Research and Development** aspects. Review and update **Project Execution Plan**, including **Change Control Procedures**. Review and update **Construction** and **Health and Safety Strategies**. |
| Sustainability Checkpoints | **Sustainability Checkpoint — 0** | **Sustainability Checkpoint — 1** | **Sustainability Checkpoint — 2** | **Sustainability Checkpoint — 3** |
| Information Exchanges (at stage completion) | **Strategic Brief.** | **Initial Project Brief.** | **Concept Design** including outline structural and building services design, associated **Project Strategies**, preliminary **Cost Information** and **Final Project Brief**. | **Developed Design**, including the coordinated architectural, structural and building services design and updated **Cost Information**. |
| UK Government Information Exchanges | Not required. | Required. | Required. | Required. |

**\*Variable task bar** – in creating a bespoke project or practice specific RIBA Plan of Work 2013 via www.ribaplanofwork.com a specific bar is selected from a number of options.

The **RIBA Plan of Work 2013** should be used solely as guidance for the preparation of detailed professional services contracts and building contracts.

**www.ribaplanofwork.com**

| 4 Technical Design | 5 Construction | 6 Handover and Close Out | 7 In Use |
|---|---|---|---|
| Prepare **Technical Design** in accordance with **Design Responsibility Matrix** and **Project Strategies** to include all architectural, structural and building services information, specialist subcontractor design and specifications, in accordance with **Design Programme**. | Offsite manufacturing and onsite **Construction** in accordance with **Construction Programme** and resolution of **Design Queries** from site as they arise. | Handover of building and conclusion of **Building Contract**. | Undertake **In Use** services in accordance with **Schedule of Services**. |
| **2013** will set out the specific tendering and procurement activities that will occur at each stage in relation to the chosen procurement route. | Administration of **Building Contract**, including regular site inspections and review of progress. | Conclude administration of **Building Contract**. | |
| or being undertaken concurrently. A bespoke **RIBA Plan of Work 2013** will clarify the stage overlaps. | The **Project Programme** will set out the specific stage dates and detailed programme durations. | | |
| planning application is to be made. | | | |
| Review and update **Sustainability, Maintenance and Operational** and **Handover Strategies** and **Risk Assessments**. Prepare and submit Building Regulations submission and any other third party submissions requiring consent. Review and update **Project Execution Plan**. Review **Construction Strategy**, including sequencing, and update **Health and Safety Strategy**. | Review and update **Sustainability Strategy** and implement **Handover Strategy**, including agreement of information required for commissioning, training, handover, asset management, future monitoring and maintenance and ongoing compilation of 'As-constructed' Information. Update **Construction** and **Health and Safety Strategies**. | Carry out activities listed in **Handover Strategy** including **Feedback** for use during the future life of the building or on future projects. Updating of **Project Information** as required. | Conclude activities listed in **Handover Strategy** including **Post-occupancy Evaluation**, review of **Project Performance, Project Outcomes** and **Research and Development** aspects. Updating of **Project Information**, as required, in response to ongoing client **Feedback** until the end of the building's life. |
| **Sustainability Checkpoint — 4** | **Sustainability Checkpoint — 5** | **Sustainability Checkpoint — 6** | **Sustainability Checkpoint — 7** |
| Completed **Technical Design** of the project. | **'As-constructed' Information**. | Updated **'As-constructed' Information**. | **'As-constructed' Information** updated in response to ongoing client **Feedback** and maintenance or operational developments. |
| Not required. | Not required. | Required. | As required. |

© RIBA

09

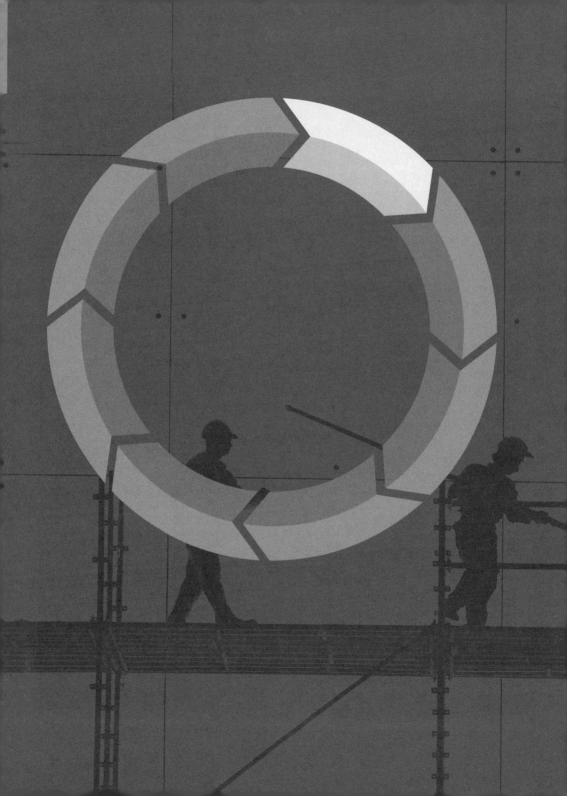

Stage 0

# Strategic
# Definition

# Chapter overview

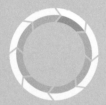

Stage 0 sets the scene for the project context. It is critical that an examination of the project's Business Case is conducted at this time. Health and safety must be part of any initial thoughts; otherwise, it might never be addressed properly in the following stages of the project.

Also during this stage, the Project Programme and significant milestones need to be established. Drafting the Project Programme and the Project Objectives, including proposals for briefing, design, construction and post-completion activities, is perhaps the most important task during this stage.

**The key coverage in this chapter is as follows:**

Get organised to deliver the Strategic Brief

The structure of health and safety in the UK

The essential regulations

Areas to be aware of within the project

Areas to be aware of outside the project

Health and safety influence and approach

Project preparation strategy in the office

What to do: Setting the Strategic Brief

Information Exchanges

# Introduction

The RIBA Plan of Work 2013 can be a powerful tool for ensuring that health and safety outcomes are delivered at every stage of the project. Consideration of the most important factors at this stage will frame how successful this will be.

Much of this chapter's content focuses on the general set-up of the health and safety environment, which, once established, will not be repeated. It is included at this point to ensure that readers have a comprehensive explanation of the issues, as if they were meeting them for the first time.

*Establishing the health and safety business case*

Setting out the health and safety sections of the Strategic Brief means aligning good practice in this area with the other Project Objectives. Establishing a strong commitment to health and safety – to ensuring that no one is exposed to harm during construction or beyond – in Stage 0 almost certainly makes projects more efficient and better organised and improves value for money.

*Strategic Brief*

As the starting point for the project, the Strategic Brief is distilled from the initial analysis – a major feature of the RIBA Plan of Work 2013. Emerging from this should be the need to emphasise a commitment to health and safety by setting out some clear goals. Successive government construction strategies have made health and safety a key topic; this is set to continue.

Health and safety principles for consideration in a Strategic Brief should include the following:

Health and safety should always be included as a headline agenda item for project meetings.

Health must be given the same status as safety.

There must be clear reporting lines and information flows between the board room and the workforce.

There is a responsibility – starting with the client, but extending to everyone in authority across the project – to ensure that any actions necessary to avoid risk will be taken throughout the project.

The focus must be on practical actions, not on complex procedures.

### Project Programme

Time and resources are the necessary ingredients for best practice in health and safety. The Project Programme must allow for adequate planning and organisation if the very best results are to be achieved. Conflicts in the Project Programme and insufficient time allowances must be avoided.

### Information Exchanges

Information Exchanges are required in the RIBA Plan of Work 2013, and are aligned with those in the UK Government's Level 2 BIM strategy. These occur at Stages 1, 2, 3 and 6, and in some cases at Stage 7, and seek to ensure that Project Information is verified and, wherever possible, is checked to ensure that the project is on track. The Information Exchanges must incorporate the relevant health and safety information at each stage. In Building Information Modelling (BIM) driven projects these exchanges will involve formatted data, allowing them to be automated. Information Exchanges ensure that the right information is being issued, the brief is being followed, overall delivery is on time and performance can be verified by the client. These are identified at the end of each chapter of this guide.

As small offices have only limited resources it is essential to have simple project procedures in place and to take advantage of free sources of information.

- Everything has to be in proportion – do not feel that health and safety reporting needs lots of words, elaborate formats or complex explanations.
- Messages are most easily understood when simply expressed.
- Learn from past conversations with the client.
- Record the project by means of a simple spreadsheet.
- Have simple templates, checklists and standard letters that require a minimum of additional detail – preferably just the project-specific information.
- Have a good understanding of legal requirements, but not obsessively so.
- Ensure you know where to look for sources of information, to save time when you need it.

## What are the Core Objectives of this stage?

The Core Objectives of the RIBA Plan of Work 2013 at Stage 0 are:

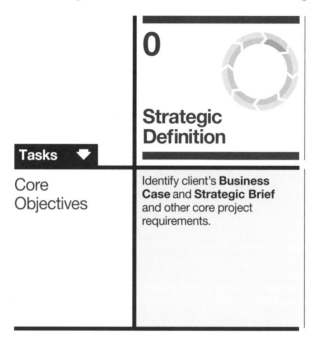

**0**

**Strategic Definition**

| Tasks ▼ | |
| --- | --- |
| Core Objectives | Identify client's **Business Case** and **Strategic Brief** and other core project requirements. |

The Core Objectives at this stage are the establishment of the client's Strategic Brief and the Business Case for the project.

At this stage it is essential to ensure the project will be well organised and properly focused. It will be necessary to take stock of the client's aspirations and initial thoughts and to organise them for best effect.

It is critical that the big-ticket items are included in the Strategic Brief. The context of health and safety within the project, the authority it is given, the clear reporting lines and the value placed on simple, practical outcomes should all be in there. It should sit well with current industry and government aspirations and, if the bar is to be raised, exceed them.

## Practice Note: Get organised to deliver the Strategic Brief

Projects must start with an organised approach, stemming from the Strategic Brief. All project team members need to have organisational ability. While most will profess to being well organised, sadly this is often not the case in reality. Getting organised is straightforward, and keeping everything legal saves time and money and allows a better service to be delivered to clients.

In the context of the RIBA Plan of Work 2013, organisational issues are best considered prior to even Stage 0. Any well-organised practice needs to keep abreast of such issues, but, once established, they require little effort to keep up to date. This starts with good information.

### Sources of information

Good sources of free information are available – subscriptions or paid-for downloads are not always necessary. A lot of free information just needs to be found and filed, and the general contents committed to memory.

The Health and Safety Executive (HSE) produces free guidance that covers the full range of health and safety, from general office, health and procedure information to project specifics. It is sensible to have copies of the HSE guides downloaded and stored in a dedicated location on the office system.

For any items of third party information you hold:

- check at least once a year that they are up to date
- do not rely on others' interpretations – always go the original versions, as any interpretations offered by others might be biased
- cross-check them against other sources to arrive at a balanced view.

### Health and safety manual

Every office, big or small, needs a health and safety manual (see page 34). This will include details on the practice's policies and procedures for health and safety, and provide basic reference material and sources of information and training. It can also be used as part of any prequalification documentation required by potential client organisations.

### Standardise responses to reduce paperwork

There are a number of common actions where having a pre-prepared standard response will save time, provide consistency and ensure you have completed what needs to be done. There will be occasions when

## Practice Note: Get organised to deliver the Strategic Brief (*continued*)

pro-forma responses will need to be changed to fit a particular project, and will have to be reviewed regularly and updated, but the time savings and consistency they give is worth it.

Examples include the following:

– letter to clients explaining their duties under the Construction (Design and Management) Regulations 2015 (CDM regulations) and asking for confirmation of receipt
– letter to contractors identifying office procedures
– risk design evaluation process and template
– risk design matrix process and template
– residual design risk evaluation template
– letters of appointment
– record sheets – for example, for recording that key stages have been completed
– guidance notes – for clients and contractors, giving clear processes to follow, or for use in prequalification to demonstrate proficiency
– case studies – examples of previous projects are always useful for explaining to clients, other consultants and project managers the practice's previous experience.

### Prequalification and health and safety

Having a prequalification document on file, already filled in with supporting practice information on health and safety, saves time and improves efficiency. Even if it is not specifically requested, this document should be included as standard in any prequalification response. The client or prequalification organisation can then ask for any further information it might require.

### Training

Keep training up to date, and always include health and safety in your programme. Look for good, engaging training material, to keep everyone interested. Keep all records up to date, so that if a client asks to see them they can be made available with a minimum of fuss and effort.

### Company structure

Every company needs to have an organogram identifying the structure of the management and showing the team responsibilities within the office. This must show roles and responsibilities and the relationships between

## Practice Note: Get organised to deliver the Strategic Brief (*continued*)

levels of hierarchy. This is a requirement of the Management of Health and Safety at Work Regulations 1999.

### Management standards

BS EN ISO 9001: 2015 and, especially, BS EN ISO 9004: 2009 are useful guides for developing the core management principles. While not directly linked to health and safety, they are good reference points for essential management behaviours and determine the fundamentals of good practice. Both are recommended reading.

### Avoiding unnecessary work

Health and safety has been given a bad name by the inappropriate use of default positions and by not being incorporated into mainstream processes. However, using a common-sense approach can significantly reduce the amount of work required:

– Extensive written health and safety processes are not necessary. As well as being time consuming, they often miss the point and have been proven to be ineffective.
– Using numerical health and safety assessments is pointless. These have been tried in the past and failed, being opinion based and offering no real benefit.
– Including a health and safety box on every drawing can result in the information shown becoming too general to be of benefit. This procedure – which is often more about showing that senior management is 'serious' about health and safety – becomes a pointless waste of time and energy as the boxes are never read or acted upon.

# The structure of health and safety in the UK

Everyone involved in a project needs to have a contextual understanding of health and safety. The Strategic Brief should adopt a robust approach to health and safety – it shouldn't be treated simply as a legislative hurdle.

UK law relating to health and safety is centred around two key principles:

I case law
I the concept 'so far as is reasonably practicable' (SFARP, defined below).

## Statutory instruments

Health and safety legislation is generally enacted through a number of statutory instruments (regulations). It is always recommended that you read the instrument that covers any particular health and safety issue, rather than just relying on a third party interpretation, to ensure you understand the actual legal requirements.

## Approved guidance

Many elements of UK law are accompanied by an approved code of practice (ACOP). While these are not legally enforceable, they are often used by the courts to settle disputes. However, there are also other sources of guidance, such as the HSE's L series documents, which give clear definitions and descriptions of legal requirements.

## Supporting standards

Some aspects of design and management are supported by British or international standards or codes of practice, or by other significant references. In particular, some parts of the Building Regulations are supported by several nested sets of relevant standards.

## Custom and practice surrounding the law

It is common for some methods to become accepted as standard practice. This becomes important when considering design risk assessment. If a long-established process is deemed to be harmful, such as controlling dust in cutting operations by damping down with water, then attempting to change such entrenched behaviour can be challenging.

## Seeking advice

The HSE is the prime agency when considering issues of risk and hazard management. Specifically, its construction team initiates legislation guidance and has enforcement powers. Whenever a question arises, it is always sensible to refer to HSE guidance, most of which is downloadable without charge. The HSE is very approachable, so any serious worries can be raised with it directly.

## How does this play out in practice?

UK law is broadly divided into civil and criminal. Most law that the designer needs to understand is civil. However, health and safety legislation – and the CDM regulations in particular – is criminal law. This has significant implications in that any action the HSE wishes to take can seriously affect the individual involved and the company they work for.

A central and significant tenet of UK legal provisions is the SFARP concept. This is applied right across the spectrum of health and safety legislation. To some this is frustrating as there is no definitive level or action that determines compliance. It is more a test of what is sensible and proportionate: would the average person have reacted in that way? This principle is deeply embedded in our legal structure.

### So far as is reasonably practicable (SFARP)

The concept of balancing the level of a risk against the measures needed to control it, in terms of money, time or trouble. Action is not needed if it would be grossly disproportionate to the level of risk.

See also www.hse.gov.uk/risk/faq.htm

Legislation is supplemented by case law. Cases that have previously come to prominence in the legal system are used as reference material: where a judgment has been made, this establishes precedence. The factors taken into account and used to determine guilt or innocence in the original case are then applied to any subsequent cases. This has effectively created a tipping point around the concept of SFARP.

Designers should always remember they are not lawyers, but they should have a good understanding both of the principles and practice of law.

### Get advice

Where you have any doubts, it is essential that you seek appropriate advice. This could be from colleagues, your professional body or your insurer or from a legal professional with experience in this area.

## The essential regulations

Many pieces of legislation have implications for health and safety, but the most significant ones are:

I The Construction (Design and Management) Regulations 2015
I The Management of Health and Safety at Work Regulations 1999
I The Workplace (Health, Safety and Welfare) Regulations 1992
I The Building Regulations 2010 (Technical Standards in Scotland)
I The Regulatory Reform (Fire Safety) Order 2005
I The Control of Asbestos Regulations 2012.

### Other regulations

It must be remembered that other important sets of regulations might have to be considered, particularly in relation to specific technical details. These can have significant implications for design and so should not be overlooked.

The HSE provides a series of guides that can be downloaded for free and used as the core reference for each of the following pieces of legislation.

### The CDM regulations

The Construction (Design and Management) Regulations 2015 are the principal regulations governing health and safety in construction. The regulations are set out to follow the natural chronology of a construction project, although they do not follow the RIBA Plan of Work stages precisely. There are specific duties and actions that the CDM regulations require, covering the design, construction and in use phases of a project – these are discussed on pages 51–62: Stage 1.

The regulations implement EU Council Directive 92/57/EEC (on temporary or mobile construction sites). One of the essential principles of this is the use of the term 'coordination and cooperation', meaning that workers and project team members should work together in every sense to ensure they minimise health and safety risks. Only by doing this can they ensure safe working between them.

Emphasis on the term 'coordination and cooperation' in previous versions of the regulations resulted in it becoming overused and misinterpreted by non-designers. Cooperation and coordination are skills that have always been required by design teams throughout the modern era. Every design team member understands the importance of these. Frequent reference to them in the directive and subsequent overemphasis by many non-designers has made them a source of irritation, frustration and inefficiency. The new approach adopted in the 2015 regulations should result in fewer misunderstandings.

Under the CDM regulations, projects over a certain size must be notified to the HSE. The process around notification of projects has not changed for many years, although the trigger points for notification have been simplified in the 2015 regulations. A project is notifiable if it will:

| require more than 30 days' continuous working and have more than 20 workers at any one time, or
| involve more than 500 person days.

### CDM and small projects

For very small projects with a domestic client and one contractor the responsibilities to work safely under the terms of the CDM regulations still apply, but with a different emphasis.

The specific roles and requirements of the CDM regulations are described throughout this guide, within the stages where they are most relevant, and a synopsis of the changes introduced in the 2015 regulations is provided at appendix 1.

### The management regulations

The Management of Health and Safety at Work Regulations 1999 ('the management regulations') identify the structure and behaviour of organisations in respect of the management of business operations. All those in positions of authority should be aware of their provisions and of the requirements that they impose on them as individuals.

HSG 65: *Managing for health and safety* shows that the provisions of these regulations are straightforward, but the team must still be alert to them.

## The workplace regulations

The Workplace (Health, Safety and Welfare) Regulations 1992 ('the workplace regulations') are now incorporated within the CDM regulations, and the majority are also covered by the Building Regulations (see appendix 2 for a detailed analysis).

L24: *Workplace health, safety and welfare. Workplace (Health, Safety and Welfare) Regulations 1992. Approved Code of Practice and guidance* is a useful source for good practice guidance.

## The Fire Safety Order

In 2005, the many elements of fire safety legislation were consolidated under the Regulatory Reform (Fire Safety) Order 2005 ('the FSO'). For designers, the most significant part of the order is the requirement to ensure that information is produced for building owners and occupants in respect of fire safety provisions. This requirement is often overlooked, but it is an essential task as building control can refuse to sign off the project until it is completed.

The FSO regulations are often overlooked in design. However, HSG 168: *Fire safety in construction* clearly identifies what is expected of the design team. The need to ensure that the design is safe from a fire perspective, under the Building Regulations, is well understood.

It is important that obligations under this legislation are reviewed during Stage 0. As the technical detail is developed during later stages, issues around fire risk and safety become more apparent. It is vital, especially for more vulnerable construction types, that the design team not only identifies the potential issues, but also offers solutions to their construction colleagues.

Design teams need to understand the requirements of the FSO and, while developing the design, discuss their implications with the client. Later, during Stage 5, the discussion will need to be picked up with the contractor.

## The Building Regulations

The original and prime objectives of the Building Regulations were health and safety. The Building Regulations 2010 (excluding Scotland) contain a wide range of complex requirements, but they still address these fundamentals.

In particular, regulation 38 requires the design team to provide fire safety information for the building in use. Failure to do so can result in the approving organisation refusing Building Regulations sign-off. It is surprising how little known this requirement is, yet failure to provide the appropriate information can open up the consultant team to liability, or even an insurance claim.

## The regulations connections

In summary, the design is expected to allow for fire safety during the build, driven by the CDM regulations and the management regulations and supported by HSE guidance. On completion adequate information must be provided as required by the CDM regulations, the FSO and regulation 38 of the Building Regulations. This can be challenging for the design team, as most of the actions and all of the authority will be vested in the contractor. Nonetheless, a team employing good practice will seek out issues that may arise during construction and ensure that the contractor and client are aware of them.

## The asbestos regulations

While asbestos has been banned from use in new projects for a very long time, it is still present in many buildings and across the built environment. The Control of Asbestos Regulations 2012 ('the asbestos regulations') are very explicit – all members of the design team should understand them and be aware of the provisions, as well as the practical implications of finding this material on site.

The HSE is again the best source of information on how to comply with the asbestos regulations: in fact, it is recommended that only HSE information is used for this purpose. Third party information is sometimes tainted by misinterpretation or overprovision.

For every project involving an existing building, an asbestos manger should be appointed and an asbestos survey conducted, with the findings made available to the whole team. Regardless of what the asbestos survey might show, everyone involved in any site visit needs to be aware that asbestos might be present on site and know what to do if they suspect they find some.

All design team members should receive regular training on asbestos, encompassing the HSE guidance. However, it is usually not necessary for them to attend asbestos awareness courses.

## Common standards

There are a number of different common standards, so it is important that it is agreed from the start which standards will be used. Agree those to be used from the start.

## Other guidance

There are many other significant regulations and supporting codes of practice. While their use might be implied in the Strategic Brief, it is common that they are not explicitly identified. The following have significant implications for the design and construction of buildings.

I The Work at Height Regulations 2005 – These regulations were introduced to control an area where many accidents occur. Any project team should understand the importance of limiting and controlling activities at height as accidents involving falls, especially on small sites, top the HSE statistics. These regulations place a duty on everyone involved on a project, but especially those in authority, to ensure workers have the correct safety equipment and the right training and are sufficiently skilled for the task.

I Control of Major Accident Hazards Regulations 2015 (COMAH) – health and welfare guidance.

I Control of Substances Hazardous to Health Regulations 2002 (as amended) (COSHH) – INDG 136 harmful substances guidance.

I Registration, Evaluation, Authorisation and Restriction of Chemicals regulation (REACH) – restricted chemicals requirements (see HSE website).

I BS 9999: 2008 *Code of practice for fire safety in the design, management and use of buildings.*

I Site Safe design guidance for fire prevention. Structural Timber Association.

I BS 8560: 2012 *Code of practice for the design of buildings incorporating safe work at height.*

I BS OHSAS 18001: 2007 *Occupational health and safety management systems. Requirements.*

# Areas to be aware of within the project

## Setting up the project

Clearly, it is impossible to identify every project-specific health and safety issue at the outset. Instead, the core principles must be established, which will form the heart of the project's Health and Safety Strategy. Initially, the team may be small, perhaps just the architect or project manager and the client.

From the start, the client must be made aware of their responsibilities for health and safety – as the instigator of the project, most of the liabilities lie with the client. Many clients are aware that their business must operate with good health and safety principles at its core. The degree of assistance needed by the client will vary considerably.

### HSE guidance

A good starting reference is HSG 150: *Health and safety in construction.* It covers every aspect of construction and clearly denotes the legal requirements and good practice. It is a highly recommended and useful reference source.

## Health and safety prequalification

Prequalification has developed into an industry all of its own. However, there is concern over the amount of bureaucracy that has arisen, due to those running prequalification schemes often having little understanding of consultants and the design team. To reduce this burden, the systems, procedures and formulas used for managing health and safety on projects can be used to support prequalification applications.

### The industry and prequalification

Prequalification in the construction industry can be a complex process. For many practices working in the private sector, prequalification is more straightforward and less bureaucratic than for those working in the public

## Guidance on procurement

The EU directive on public sector procurement stipulates the format and process to be used for team appointments across a large section of the market. This is a complex area and cannot be covered here. There are several excellent guides on the subject that can help to clarify the process, including:

*A Practical Guide to Public Procurement,* by Abby Semple (2015).

sector where there are many more formulas to be applied and gateways to be negotiated.

### PAS 91: 2013 – the government's preferred prequalification format

PAS 91: 2013 *Construction prequalification questionnaires* seeks to standardise prequalification processes. Its standardised questionnaires have been drawn up to allow applicants to fill them in once and use them many times across many projects, with the aim of cutting down on effort and repetition. Unfortunately, it has not yet gained the degree of use hoped for by the HSE. (At the time of going to press, PAS 91 is up for revision.)

### SSIP helping reduce bureaucracy

Often, clients will appoint a specialist to handle their prequalification process. Safety Schemes in Procurement (SSIP) seeks to align the large number of organisations that offer this service for clients. The group, which is independent of but encouraged by the HSE, provides a 'deemed to satisfy' route for applicants, ie membership of one health and safety prequalification scheme provides membership of any other within the SSIP.

## Safety Schemes in Procurement

Information on the scheme can be found at: www.ssip.org.uk

## Early client approaches

### The regular client

A regular client will be the easiest type of client to engage with. They will already have an understanding of the relevant legislation, and will often have their own bespoke procedures. Because they know the territory they will be unlikely to adopt a casual approach to the application of procedures or to shortcut formal dutyholder requirements.

Before an initial meeting, it is a good idea to ask to see a copy of the client's health and safety procedures. Work through these and highlight areas of good practice for discussion, and identify any gaps that need addressing.

### The one-off client

A one-off client will usually need to be helped through the process. Such clients will usually be involved with a business and be familiar with legal structures and processes, so will just need help to understand the specific regulations that apply to their project.

It can be helpful to organise a workshop to discuss health and safety. This can help the client to understand what they need to do, and what else can be done throughout the project to achieve high standards.

If this type of client is a common source of business, it may be worth producing a simple guide to explain the process and the client duties.

### CDM and the client

The client, being the instigator of the project, has ultimate responsibility for compliance with the CDM regulations. Under the 2015 regulations, even a domestic client (someone who is undertaking work to their own home) has responsibilities. There is a clear set of actions that the client must discharge.

## The domestic client

Under the 2015 CDM regulations, a domestic client now has responsibilities for health and safety, bringing the UK into line with the EU directive on the implementation of minimum safety and health requirements at construction sites.

For a domestic client employing one contractor, the client duties are transferred to the contractor. These duties are very limited – effectively no more than the contractor would otherwise have undertaken.

For a domestic client employing more than one contractor, one of those contractors will need to be identified as the 'principal contractor'; that contractor will then take on the client duties. This will occur automatically if the client does not formally appoint a principal contractor. On a project where the principal contractor assumes the client duties, then a 'principal designer' needs to work with the contractor as if it were the client.

Additionally, the client can appoint a principal designer to assume the client duties, or this is assumed to have happened if a principal contractor is not in place, although this arrangement needs to be in writing. However, the client's responsibility cannot be transferred.

### Early engagement with domestic clients

- Provide domestic clients with a standard information pack.
- Ensure that anything that is agreed is confirmed in writing.
- Refer domestic clients to the guidance prepared by the HSE.
- Construction Industry Training Board (CITB) guidance for domestic clients is also available.

### Health and safety and the Strategic Brief

Health and safety must be part of the Project Objectives and so it is important that it is addressed as part of the Strategic Brief. The health and safety aspirations developed with increasing detail through Stages 0, 1 and 2 do not have to be complex or lengthy to be effective. They do, however, have to be developed with the total support of the client and the team members as they are appointed.

A typical Strategic Brief might consider the following health and safety aspirations:

I   Health and safety will be given due prominence across all parts of the project.
I   The 'principles of prevention' will be followed at all times.
I   The project will seek to achieve a zero harm status for everyone involved.
I   The project will focus on outcomes rather than bureaucracy.
I   Everyone is responsible for ensuring the Health and Safety Strategy is applied at all times.
I   Health will be treated with the same emphasis and attention as safety.
I   Cooperation and communication will extend across the whole project team.

### Raising the bar

Health and safety has come a long way in the past 20 years. However, on average, one person is killed per week in the UK on a construction site, and around 13,000 die each year from construction-related ill health. There is a long way to go before these statistics can be consigned to history. Employing good practice wherever possible is obviously a good start – and it is obviously good business, as it will result in a project achieving more than just regulatory compliance.

Throughout this guide there is an emphasis on good practice, with examples of practical solutions and ideas of where exemplar practice can be applied. Many clients now expect this approach and increasingly they are asking design and construction teams to deliver by raising the bar on each successive project.

## Areas to be aware of outside the project

### Changes in legislation

At the start of any project it is important to ensure that systems are in place to check for and flag up any changes to the regulatory regime. These might include changes in:

I financial/accounting rules
I planning legislation
I Building Regulations
I HSE guidance.

## Feedback from previous projects

Best practice is often developed though applying Feedback gained from completed projects – by taking what was learned on one project and using it to enhance the next. In the past it has often been difficult to revisit projects once they enter the 'in use' phase unless there is a problem. The RIBA Plan of Work 2013 recognises the importance of understanding whether the building functions as intended and includes Post-occupancy Evaluation and review of Project Outcomes as key support tasks at Stage 7: In Use. The Feedback gained here can be vital in setting up the next project and for improving the approach.

In terms of health and safety, key questions to ask when reviewing a project would include:

I Did your initial briefing of the client in respect of health and safety and subsequent actions produce good outcomes?
I Is there anything that could have been done better or explained more clearly?

### The design process

The design process is often difficult to review in detail, as so many interactions occur. However, standout moments or significant issues, good or bad, need to be identified and considered either as areas where improvements can be made or as successes to be built upon. When reviewing the approach used for design development, could a different route have been used, which would have arrived at the same outcome, but in a better way?

### Review the project 'as it went to site'

It is helpful to assess the quality of the health and safety information generated before Stage 5 (see page 146: Stage 4):

I Did the information reflect the important actions?
I Were all, or at least most, of the health and safety issues identified and addressed?
I Were any remaining issues clearly identified to the contractor?

### In use and beyond

There is a responsibility to ensure that a completed building is safe to use and maintain. Many newly completed projects will use a 'Soft Landings' methodology, which can help (see page 190: Stage 6). Health and safety under the CDM regulations is the one area where there is a legal obligation in this respect.

There is also an obligation to ensure that any potential risks that might arise at the end of the life of the building – during demolition or refurbishment – are recorded in the health and safety file. If the building has been constructed using mainstream techniques, this will not produce any issues.

## Health and safety influence and approach

Every design team member will bring clarity and professional guidance to the project at all stages. This is especially important at the beginning. But everybody involved in the project should understand both the importance and desirability of ensuring there is a focused, structured and properly delivered approach to health and safety.

### Around the site

Part of the Stage 0 discussions with the client will be about site characteristics. When appraising a selection of sites, consider the health and safety perspective during the initial appraisals.

The Site Information selection should address the following features:

I access characteristics for Construction and In Use phases
I services and infrastructure, both existing and proposed
I natural features and hazards
I contamination.

These are discussed in Stage 1: see pages 68–73.

## Project preparation strategy in the office

It is critical that the office is properly prepared and has appropriate systems in place. If standard systems have been set up, they will make starting a new project straightforward and minimise errors.

These systems should just be part of any general office system. However, as they are ultimately subject to sanctions under criminal law – the CDM regulations – they need to be relatively secure and constantly and consistently applied.

### Health and safety manual

Every company and practice should have a health and safety manual. Indeed, this is a legal requirement for all but the smallest practice. The manual should be your central resource for all things related to health and safety. This should be structured around some basic elements and set out to do a number of jobs.

First, it needs to cover policies and procedures. It should have clear examples of how these are applied. These examples should reference the RIBA Plan of Work and show what is required overall and for each stage. Second, it needs to be a reference source for staff, providing clear information on all activities. Third, it needs to be available for external reference, perhaps by clients as part of their prequalification processes. The manual could also include information on fire precautions and other responsibilities. Formatting a single document to perform several roles results in economy of effort, and means there will only be one source to keep up to date.

The health and safety manual should include the following:

I a guide to all sources of information
I written copies of all health and safety policies: to be used for reference or as stand-alone documents
I the company structure (organogram)
I training and skills policies: including training programmes and CPD procedures (training records should be kept separately)
I procedures for health and safety within the office: eg emergency escape routes, equipment briefings for new staff

- procedures for health and safety outside the office: eg travelling to sites and other offices, travelling aboard, emergencies
- project health and safety procedures (including CDM): to be applied to all projects, covering client briefings, other consultants, team working, Project Information etc
- plan of work: stage-by-stage health and safety actions
- copies of relevant legislation
- worked examples and templates
- guidance notes.

When compiling a health and safety manual, base everything on HSE advice (see page 227: Further reading), use a simple structure and keep it simple and clear. The manual must be updated annually, or when significant changes in the law occur.

## What to do: setting the Strategic Brief

Stage 0 is all about defining the Strategic Brief for the project. It is important that health and safety aspirations are included as an integral part of the brief from the start. The following advice will be applicable to any project at this stage.

### It's never too early to get prepared

Stage 0 is all about preparation: the importance of being prepared cannot be emphasised enough. Given the right preparation, establishing the Strategic Brief becomes focused and efficient. The office systems may comprise several different approaches in format and media. The format can be based around good practice or ISO 9001, or perhaps experience from previous projects. The media can range from simple paper-based to fully integrated electronic systems. Irrespective, there must be a clear understanding of what approach is needed by the client, the team and, if necessary, the regulator, and that it must be consistent and easily replicated.

### Inform the client

The most important relationships in any project are with the client and the contractor. Clients can range from complete novices to experienced campaigners. Their level of experience needs to be established and your communications and advice tailored to match. Whatever the client's experience, they must be informed of their CDM duties. This is best done in writing, which can be included in the pack of information confirming the commission. This would ideally be a separate enclosure to keep the administration simple, and best practice would involve asking the client to respond in writing.

### Construction insight

Early engagement with a source of construction insight is always recommended. However, this is not always possible. In order for the contractor's input to start well in later stages it will be necessary to have the Project Information, especially for health and safety, organised and available, with the necessary focus on construction-related issues. Some consider this so important as to recommend the appointment of a contractor in an advisory capacity. If this is to be adopted it needs early consideration.

Construction knowledge brings expertise to the situation and perhaps offers solutions. In a design and build situation it is essential that a clear set of CDM information is available prior to novation (or a switch) if the project is being handed over to the contractor's design team (see page 48: Stage 1).

### Project-specific issues

Any Project Information should focus on project-specific issues – the contractor can be expected to undertake standard construction activities without specific directions. Where, however, the requirements are not routine, a clear explanation of what has been designed is needed. The information must offer at least one practical and safe method for construction. On complex or unusual projects, it may be necessary to involve the contractor when developing the construction sequencing. These issues need to be factored into the brief development.

A balance between practical issues and aesthetics is needed. Too often, poor communication from both sides stops progress: compromise and understanding must be the right approach.

## Information Exchanges

Information Exchanges required for Stage 0 are as follows:

I  at stage completion: the Strategic Brief
I  for UK Government projects: not required.

## The Construction Commitments

The Strategic Forum for Construction's Construction Commitments addressed six areas of performance. The commitment and targets for health and safety were:

Health and safety is integral to the success of any project, from design and construction to subsequent operation and maintenance.

*2010 target*
- Reduce the incidence rate of fatal and major injury accidents by 10% year on year from 2000 levels.
- Reduce the incidence rate of cases of work-related ill health by 20% from 2000 levels.

*2012 target*
- 10% reduction year on year in the incidence rate of fatal and major injuries from 2010 levels.
- 50% increase in projects offering a route to occupational health support from 2008 level.
- 30% increase from 2007 level of micro-SMEs and SMEs taking up H&S training and education at an organisational level.

New commitments are being drawn up to build on the progress made to date.

## Chapter summary                                    0

Stage 0 is the stage-setting period. This is when experience gained from past projects is gathered together, and when preparations are made to ensure that the new project will deliver everything that is expected. It is also the time when the health and safety position is established and the health and safety aspirations formulated.

| Understand where the project development should be.
| Use as many tips and ideas as you can find.
| Ensure the whole office is prepared and knows what is needed.
| Do not rush into any quick or client-pressured decisions.
| Make sure the client is aware of their legal obligations.
| Do not be tempted to adopt poor practice.

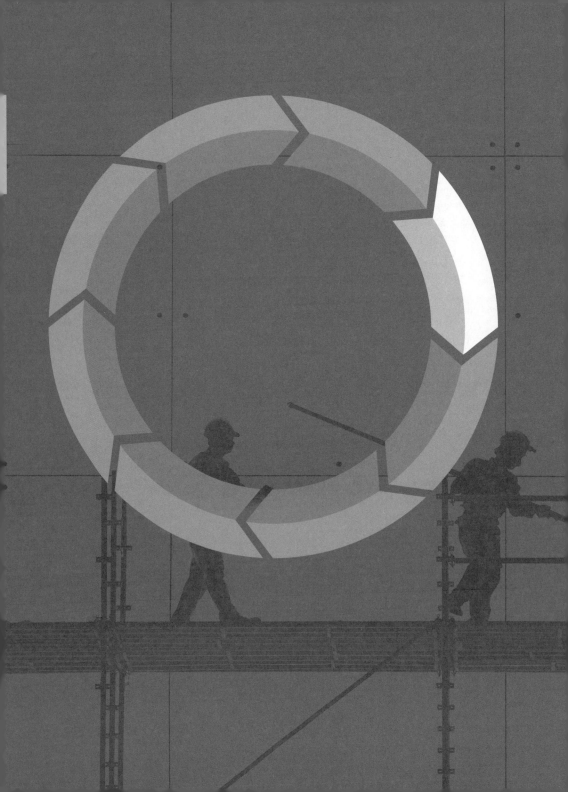

# Preparation
and Brief

# Chapter overview

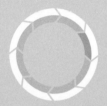

Stage 1 builds on the Strategic Brief developed in Stage 0. This is when the client's Project Outcomes must be fully woven into the Initial Project Brief and the design team selected for Stage 2.

Key areas to be covered are Quality Objectives, desired Project Outcomes, Sustainability Aspirations and Project Budget. A critical element will be the review of Site Information and the completion of any Feasibility Studies.

The RIBA Plan of Work 2013 also highlights the importance of the Project Roles Table and the Contractual Tree. As the number of team appointments grows, these become essential to ensuring the project team is suitable for the project and that team members' Schedules of Services are properly coordinated. At this stage a Design Responsibility Matrix, linked to the Project Execution Plan, and the Communication and Technology Strategies should also be developed. The latter require agreement over which technologies, common standards and forms of communication will be used on the project. These will all involve health and safety considerations.

Additional considerations during this stage include developing the Handover Strategy, to ensure there will be a smooth transition at Stage 6, after construction is complete.

Project Risk Assessments should also be drawn up at this stage (these should not be confused with health and safety risk assessments).

When developing the health and safety aspirations of the Initial Project Brief, consideration should be given to appointing a health and safety adviser. A suitably experienced architect or designer can undertake this role, but there are also independent specialists, who can be extremely valuable and offer a wider insight than would otherwise be available.

**The key coverage in this chapter is as follows:**

Project Objectives

Procurement and health and safety

CDM considerations at Stage 1

Assembling the project team

Site Information

Project Execution Plan

Handover Strategy

Risk assessments

Information Exchanges

# Introduction

A large number of important actions occur at this stage. This chapter identifies how to implement them and how best to ensure they are understood by the client and the team. It is at this stage that the health and safety aspirations need to be fleshed out, ahead of preparing the Health and Safety Strategy at Stage 2. Unfortunately, good intentions can start to be sidelined, because they are thought not to impact on time and money.

*From Stage 0*

It is important to take full advantage of the Stage 0 preparations.

Make sure the health and safety aspirations have been developed and are in place.

Apply experience gained from your previous projects and, if possible, your client's.

Ensure everyone is content with the legal and practical objectives.

Take note of possible site issues.

## What are the Core Objectives of this stage?

The Core Objectives of the RIBA Plan of Work 2013 at Stage 1 are:

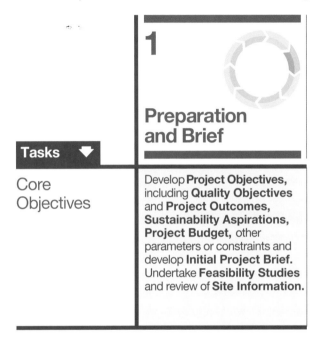

The Core Objectives at this stage focus on preparing the Initial Project Brief, which includes developing the Project Objectives, Quality Objectives, Project Outcomes, Sustainability Aspirations and Project Budget and considering other parameters or constraints. Feasibility Studies are undertaken during this stage, and Site Information reviewed.

It is the time to ensure that everything that will be needed is in place, including the Schedule of Services and the Design Responsibility Matrix, and that key Project Strategies have been prepared, particularly the Handover Strategy and Project Execution Plan. Focusing on the site and site requirements is also key at this time.

## Project Objectives

The Initial Project Brief needs to contain specific references to health and safety. This brief will cover a wide range of subjects and so it is often easy for the health and safety elements to be overshadowed.

### The health and safety perspective

- Ensure high standards throughout, enabled by good design.
- Strive for a zero-harm record throughout the project.
- Ensure all processes follow the prescribed path.
- Identify and review any near misses from previous projects.
- Consider health as well as safety.
- Do not accept second best.

### Consider the project 'in use' from the start

Remember that Practical Completion is not the end of the story. It is essential that, as the design starts to emerge, there is a focus on the completed project, and that this is reflected in the Initial Project Brief. Whatever the building, facility or asset, it will be used, cleaned, maintained and, eventually, demolished. The emerging design must provide for these activities to be entirely safe. Simply put, provide a finished building that presents minimal risk to users and maintenance staff. Feedback from previous projects will be particularly valuable in planning for Stage 7: In Use.

### Quality Objectives can support health and safety

When setting the Quality Objectives, health and safety can be overlooked. However, there are many examples of projects where a focus on quality has led to the delivery of exemplary health and safety outcomes. In short, ensure you maintain high quality across the project and this will deliver high levels of health and safety.

The quality of coordination is particularly important. High-quality design coordination will ensure that all components and building operations fit together as intended. There will be little left to chance, and therefore few unintended hazards, especially arising from unseen complexities, to cause harm. Controlling this aspect can have good results right across the project. This is about management that is efficient and organised, design that is comprehensive and buildable, and details that do not create harmful situations during construction or in use.

## Project Objectives need to be clearly identified

Ensuring that the Project Objectives, the end results, are well established and understood will give the team focus and direction. The project team members will understand where the project is intended to be going and be able to work towards the end goal.

Project Objectives could include specific health and safety objectives, such as:

I  stated limits on health and safety statistics, eg so many person hours without injury
I  stated health improvements for all workers during the project
I  provision of on-site occupational health facilities or periodic visits
I  creation of healthy environments during construction, with stated limits or objectives
I  limiting the impact of construction work on the health and safety of occupants and people in areas adjacent to the site.

## Sustainability Aspirations can have an impact on health and safety

There is a clear connection between a project's Sustainability Aspirations and its health and safety outcomes. One can aid the other. However, while top-level considerations, targets and legislation have been ever present, sustainability has struggled to be seen as relevant. Boardrooms may have become full of sustainability directors, and many companies now publish sustainability policies, but progress has been slow on the ground. Embedding sustainability criteria within the whole range of construction has been difficult; there is an obvious focus on energy conservation, but even this is driven by regulation, not by philosophical change. Other aspects have taken much longer to achieve any practical prominence.

In many ways the same is true of health and safety – having been driven by regulation, some principles have taken years to be implemented in practice. It is true that hard hats, high-visibility vests etc are rarely missing from site these days. But ensuring all designs reflect good practice and that all health issues are addressed on site is still to be achieved, and design has its part to play.

## Sustainability introduces new risks

Some sustainability requirements are changing how buildings are designed, and quite rightly. For example, roofs now often include energy collection or rainwater harvesting systems, and elevations might incorporate passive shading or brise soleil. These elements are often complex assemblies and, as they are currently not very common, can lead to unforeseen problems on site. The Initial Project Brief, through the Sustainability Aspirations, should outline any requirements for sustainable technologies, so that they can be reviewed during the course of the design development. This will ensure that the implications of adopting these technologies can be clearly explained to the project team, and that the installed applications will be as harm-free as possible.

## Maintenance and cleaning considerations

From the start the brief must include provisions for any maintenance and cleaning operations in the completed building to be undertaken safely, and these must be kept under constant review as part of the design development phase. This is not always easy due to the conflicting demands of project design, but it needs to be a solid focus of consideration at this stage. Any design decisions made at this stage will influence the Maintenance and Operational Strategy prepared during Stage 2.

If necessary for clarity, call in specialist advice during critical brief development periods, for example to establish that:

I  zoning and site arrangements are achievable, and
I  potential storey heights can be accommodated.

These examples indicate how this issue can affect the initial design development. Some clients understand and demand such attention to detail, but others might not be aware that it needs to be considered at this stage.

### Project Budget and possible conflicts with health and safety

When setting the Project Budget (as part of the Project Objectives), it needs to be acknowledged that health and safety, like other core aspects, is not optional. Elements of design or equipment provision that affect health and safety can often be seen as optional, and passing on the responsibility, or indeed the problem, as acceptable, if not normal, practice. Having different budgets for capital expenditure (CAPEX) and operational expenditure (OPEX) can reinforce this view: safety equipment can be omitted from the design to make savings in the CAPEX budget, but if the OPEX budget does not permit adequate expenditure on health and safety provision, then operatives could be left maintaining an unsafe building. So-called 'value engineering' exercises also often lead to design elements intended to provide an acceptable level of safety being removed on the grounds of cost.

At this stage the Project Budget must provide for health and safety in balance with everything else. This can include provision for physical elements, such as rooftop barriers, or procedural elements, such as allowing enough money for survey work or to ensure that the right size of team will be available for certain tasks.

## Procurement and health and safety

Project procurement will commence during this stage. Any procurement activities – both in terms of the procurement strategy for the project overall and the procurement of individual goods and services by the design team and/or contractor – must include consideration of health and safety.

In procuring services, it is essential to ensure that the expertise, skills and attention needed to cover health and safety aspects will be present. This can often be overlooked in the selection process.

In procurement of a design team this is even more critical. There is a wide range of approaches to choose from, depending on the project size and complexity and the contract form to be used, but one common health and safety concern. The procurement process on most projects leads to change, either because performance specifications are turned into actual products, specified products are unavailable or are thought to be too expensive, or other factors intervene.

Even a small change in a specification or the purchasing of a substitute material for the one the design team has identified could have serious implications. Any documents, drawings or specifications (or electronic equivalents) should contain information on the health and safety attributes that the design team consider important. This will make clear to the procurement team which elements are critical for health and safety and which could be changed without reducing the health and safety quality.

The team therefore can be alert to the issues that may crop up, which will be different for each sector and vary depending on the procurement regime. A proactive approach can be adopted. This can flag the key health and safety areas as procurement goes ahead and point out the key principle that, no matter what the change, health and safety cannot be omitted.

## The range of procurement options

For any project there will be a range of procurement routes that could be chosen. These are addressed in the RIBA Plan of Work in a variable task bar. The benefits and weaknesses of the different options should be considered for each project. The project team should agree which route will be used as early as possible, so that the Project Roles Table and Contractual Tree can be prepared before the end of Stage 1.

### Traditional contract

Most in the construction industry will be aware of traditional procurement, especially at the smaller end of the market, where this is still the most common route. This form of procurement is centred on a fully detailed and specified set of information (produced at Stage 4), with the design team in authority throughout.

Adopting a traditional route should by definition mean that health and safety risks are controlled by the design team, and that the whole team will be well aware of issues that can go wrong or cause harm and take steps to prevent them occurring. As a result, much more onus is placed on the design team.

### Design and build contract

Design and build forms of contract have largely taken over the medium- and large-scale sectors of the market. The client's team produces a set of Employer's Requirements (typically at Stage 3). The contractor's team then prepares a set of Contractor's Proposals based on these documents, which it uses as the basis of its tender for the project. If the contractor is awarded the Building Contract, it completes the design and uses its skills to deliver the project.

The implication of this route for health and safety is that there is a disconnect halfway through the design process. The client's team need to be clear what the design implications are and what risks remain to be addressed. They need to have a comprehensive handover of this material to the contractor's design team, who will use this information to develop the design and the pre-construction information. The advantage is that the contractor's team can also develop the construction phase plan and, in parallel, the health and safety file as part of the Health and Safety Strategy (see pages 149–151: Stage 4). The contractor may adopt the client's original team, which will bring comprehensive knowledge of the project.

It will be critical to ensure that the Health and Safety Strategy remains in place after handover. It is also necessary for all information to be clear, especially if it is to be handed between the teams, and to establish who has authority over which parts of the design and the means of resolving any risk areas.

A variant is the two-stage form of design and build, where selection is made on the basis of an outline bid, which is then further refined in a second stage. The implications for health and safety are broadly the same as for the one-stage form.

### Management contract

Management forms of contract involve the client's design team developing a design and the contractor joining the project team quite early on, between Stages 2 and 3. The contractor then manages the project, organising it into packages that are let as separate subcontracts. While management contracting is known for achieving quality and exactly what the client requires, it is less popular than it was, as costs tend to exceed budgets.

Having a joined-up team present for nearly the whole project offers benefits for health and safety. The client may be much more hands on, and their authority can strongly influence behaviour, especially on site. However, the fragmented work packages can result in poor communication and a division of responsibilities. It is therefore difficult to enforce an overall strategy, unless a strong client and management team is in place. Also, the design team can feel one step behind, which can lead to unmanaged activities with an increase in risk.

With this form of contracting, activities are more diverse and are often out of sequence in comparison with traditional contracting. Therefore, it can be quite difficult to anticipate where risks might develop. The link between the design team and the team managing and controlling site operations is often tenuous at best, which can result in opportunities for risk reduction through design being lost.

## Considerations for small and large projects

Most small projects use the traditional procurement route. Often the Building Contract, once let to a contractor, will involve the architect (perhaps in discussion with the contractor) in tendering significant parts of the project. Most of the time the tendering will be on the basis of full information, so there will be little left to change during tender acceptance.

In the case of specialist subcontractor items, however, such as roofing or glazing, these are let as self-contained items. Contractors' submissions may contain subtle but significant differences from the tender documents, and care should be taken to tease out any issues that may increase risk. While the originator of the change may well be responsible under the law, any accident occurring due to the change will reflect badly on those in authority on the project. There have been several accidents involving groundworks and foundation underpinning or basement construction that fall into this category. The work, while part of a larger project, was let as a 'self-contained' operation to excavate the basement and a lack of expertise led to a collapse with fatal consequences.

On larger projects the tier-two and supply chain procurement routes can be complex and become remote from the design team. At the extreme, procurement activities may be handled entirely by another team, normally under the control of the main contractor. In these circumstances the design team need to explain clearly where there are any health and safety issues and how they must be controlled. As procurement advances there is almost certainly a need for the principal designer and principal contractor to review all the packages that have been let and specifically analyse the details for any areas where changes have resulted in an increase in risk.

## CDM considerations at Stage 1

At Stage 1 the structure of the project team will become more defined (see page 62). The project team members will be assigned their various roles, each of which has specific duties under the CDM regulations. These duties will extend through the course of the project (see figure 1.1), so getting the team structure right at this stage is essential.

### The client

The client must ensure that the basic provisions of the CDM regulations are in place. Most clients normally employ a consultant as a first step. They in turn have a duty to ensure the client is advised of their responsibilities under the regulations. Specifically, the client as the instigator of the project has overall responsibility to ensure everything is done according to the regulations. Any failure to address their requirements is legally the client's responsibility. While many clients will want to appoint a specialist health and safety adviser or others to undertake the work, the responsibility cannot be transferred. The client remains ultimately responsible at all times, but will rely on their team for advice.

Clients must ensure that:

- they have a properly experienced team in place
- there are adequate resources and time to undertake the project
- the work will be done in accordance with the CDM regulations.

### The designer

The HSE is clear that designers have a strong impact on early decisions, and that these can fundamentally affect the health and safety aspects of a project. The early influence and engagement of designers is therefore important.

Furthermore, as these decisions are developed, the designer is best placed to ensure that the health and safety aspects of the design are not compromised. The designer will have to juggle the many parameters as the design develops; it is their ability to keep the conflicting issues in balance, and ultimately generate a solution, that makes them ideal to be at the centre of pre-construction considerations of health and safety.

| Project role | 0 Strategic Definition | 1 Preparation and Brief | 2 Concept Design | 3 Developed Design |
|---|---|---|---|---|
| Client | Possible need<br>Project idea<br>Business Case | Strategy<br>Business plan<br>Initial team appointed | Review<br>Design team appointed | Review<br>Ensure strategy in place |
| Principal designer (PD) | Possible appointment<br>Use information from Post-occupancy Evaluation (POE) Stage 7<br>Formulate strategy | Appointment<br>Assemble Site Information<br>Start pre-construction plan<br>H&S file start | Issue form F10<br>Manage information<br>Ensure team working together<br>Develop H&S file | Ensure team work together, coordinate and cooperate<br>Manage information and H&S file |
| Designer | Possible appointment | Possible appointment<br>Liaise with PD | Work with others in team to minimise risk<br>Record information | Work with others in team to minimise risk<br>Record information |
| Principal contractor (PC) | | | | Possible advisory role<br>Help with buildability |
| Contractor | | | | Possible advisory role for specialist, eg curtain walling |
| Existing Site Information | | | | |
| Pre-construction information | | | | |
| Construction phase plan | | | | |
| Health and safety file | | | | |

Notes:
1: For general guidance only – for details see the relevant sections.
2: Subject to the appointments and contract strategy the client employs.
3: In Stage 6, options 1 and 2 are: 1. PD appointment continues to handover; 2. If PD appointment finishes earlier.

*Figure 1.1   Key actions under the CDM regulations*

| 4 Technical Design | 5 Construction | 6 Handover and Close Out | 7 In Use |
|---|---|---|---|
| Review feedback from team<br><br>PC appointed | Use design team for feedback<br><br>PC review | Take ownership<br><br>Review completion | Feedback<br><br>Fit out?<br><br>In Use review |
| PD role may finish; hand over H&S file to PC<br><br>If not, help with ongoing design | Design development continues if still on design team<br><br>Updating information and H&S file continues | 1. Prepare and hand over H&S file<br><br>Ensure 'As-constructed' Information is available | If still on project, collate POE information? |
| Work with others in team to minimise risk<br><br>Record information | Role finishes or decreases<br><br>If involved, as Stage 4 | Ensure information for H&S file and design is handed to PD | POE review<br><br>Feed back information for Stage 0 appointment |
| Appointment.<br><br>Pre-construction plan<br><br>Tender submissions<br><br>Review risks | Mobilise<br><br>Start on site<br><br>Welfare first<br><br>Liaise with PD | 2. Prepare and hand over H&S file<br><br>Ensure 'As-constructed' Information is available | May take part in POE if client requires |
| Tender preparation<br><br>Liaise on risk reduction | Possible advisory role for specialist, eg curtain walling | Add to 'As-constructed' Information and hand H&S file to PC | |

4: The horizontal arrows indicate periods where the specified information is being developed and collated and should be continuously kept up to date.
5: The vertical arrows indicate where part or all of the information should be used to develop a further area.

The HSE clearly acknowledges that in tackling all the issues involved, residual risks will remain in designs. These need to be identified and, if possible, sensible solutions for their neutralisation developed, but as a very minimum they must be explained to those on site or those who will use the building.

### The principal designer

In 2015 the CDM regulations introduced the new role of principal designer. For projects where there is more than one contractor, there is a requirement to appoint a principal designer and, in due course, a principal contractor.

Some flexibility is allowed in the timing of a principal designer's appointment. The principal designer should be appointed 'as early as is practicable'. However, until the Project Objectives have been determined, it may be difficult to identify who should be appointed to this role. The appointment can be made at any time from inception of the project until just before the start of work on site, however the latter is not recommended.

As soon as a designer is appointed to the project (which will ideally be for the start of Stage 2), if they are the first designer to be appointed, they may also be appointed as the principal designer.

The principal designer must ensure that the client understands their responsibilities and that the team work together in a structured and coordinated fashion. The principal designer is also responsible for ensuring

### Principal designer

A new role in the 2015 CDM regulations, the principal designer is:

- appointed by the client in writing on projects with more than one contractor
- a member of the design team
- a designer or designers – a person or organisation – that prepares designs and/or specifies products for use in construction and has control over the pre-construction phase of the project (not just the health and safety elements)
- an individual or organisation with sufficient skills, knowledge and experience to carry out the role.

that information on health and safety matters is gathered throughout the design period and handed over to the client at the end of the project.

An architect acting as principal designer may also have duties as a designer in relation to the architectural design of the project (see figure 1.2). It is also important to note that the duties of the principal designer are governed by the concept of 'so far as is reasonably practicable' (SFARP).

### Insurance for designers as principal designer

There have been concerns about the need for insurance for those taking on the principal designer role. Regrettably, some architects have gained the impression that insurance is either difficult to get or is a reason for not taking up the role. However, feedback from the major insurance providers suggests the opposite.

Any designer or practice with professional indemnity insurance that is up to date and meets the criteria for the role can be clear that insurance is not a barrier. The role is part of the business activities for the profession and must be addressed to avoid risk as with any other area. A practitioner needs to inform their insurance provider in writing that they are increasing their business scope. Of course, anyone taking on the role needs to discuss its implications with their insurance provider.

### Notifying the client

The principal designer must make the client aware of their duties under the CDM regulations. Repeat clients or large organisations acting as clients will probably be aware of their duties. However, it is the responsibility of the principal designer to ensure this is actually the case.

It is recommended that the principal designer sends the client a formal letter confirming their appointment to the role. This should be a separate communication, so that it can be filed independently. The letter should then spell out the client's duties and identify the requirements placed on the client by the CDM regulations. It should also ask for confirmation that the contents have been received and understood. The letter and the confirmation are then placed on file and added to the documentation that will be handed over at completion.

| Project role | 0 Strategic Definition | 1 Preparation and Brief | 2 Concept Design | |
|---|---|---|---|---|
| Lead designer (LD) | Early appointment makes sure team structure and management in place<br><br>Early adviser to client<br><br>Ensures strategy on key project elements in place<br><br>May help with team appointments<br><br>Sets scene for whole project | Collates information and ensures coordination of project structure, Feasibility Studies and emerging design concept<br><br>In authority over design and design team<br><br>Will advise on specialists required | Organises and leads design team meetings<br><br>Liaises with construction team if appointed early<br><br>Ensures information is circulated across team<br><br>Ensures information is coordinated across team | |
| Principal designer (PD) | Early appointment preferable<br><br>Could be at same time as lead designer | Ensures client understands their CDM responsibilities<br><br>Collates pre-construction information, mostly existing before the project<br><br>Starts pre-construction information<br><br>Starts H&S file<br><br>Starts team communication | Ensures team coordinate and cooperate<br><br>Helps with form F10 issue<br><br>Ensures risk analysis is in place and comprehensive<br><br>Extracts information from general information for H&S purposes | |
| Notes | Could logically be the same person or organisation | Main actions: Very little additional activity between LD and PD | Main actions: A focus on H&S risk reduction<br><br>H&S client assistance<br><br>Extract H&S information | |

*Figure 1.2   Comparison of the principal designer and lead designer roles*

| 3 Developed Design | 4 Technical Design | 5 Construction |
|---|---|---|
| Actions as Stage 2 plus liaison with contractor team, specialist subcontractors and suppliers<br><br>Ensures design team are undertaking coordinated design development<br><br>Ensures all information and communication across team is clear and robust | Actions as Stage 3 plus ensure detail remains coordinated<br><br>Ensures planning and Building Regulations approvals applied for and are being progressed<br><br>Ensures design team information is issued to the construction team<br><br>Ensures any external information requirements are addressed | Liaises with the contractor to ensure information flow is maintained<br><br>Engages and assists with changes on site |
| Ensures team engage with management of H&S aspects<br><br>Collates pre-construction information<br><br>Establishes and updates H&S file<br><br>Reviews designs across the team | As Stage 3 plus development of relevant details of cleaning and maintenance<br><br>If appointment finishing, makes sure there is a comprehensive handover | As Stage 4 plus, if still appointed, makes sure ongoing design work is reviewed and added to information records |
| Main actions: Ensure PD role activities are very clear<br><br>If coming to an end, spell out in writing | Main actions: Ensure position is clear if PD finishing | Main actions: Could be employed by the contractor |

## Letter to client confirming their duties under the CDM regulations

Dear Sir <Client>

Subject: Project <Name, number and reference>

**General duty of care** <paragraph optional>

In all building projects there are many legal requirements that may have an impact on them. Under a general duty of care as the Designer we feel that it is important that we should alert you, as our Client, of this matter. We suggest that you make further enquiries with your legal advisers to ensure that you fully understand the implications of such legislation on your project. Please note, however, that we are not offering such advice in this letter.

**CDM Designer's duty to inform**

We have a specific duty under the CDM Regulations 2015 (regulation 9). This duty requires us to ensure the Client is made aware of his position under the Regulations as soon as we are able to. This letter is issued to discharge that duty and in doing so we would draw your attention to some of the actions required by the Client:

- Appoint a Principal Designer.
- Provide information on Health and Safety issues to the Principal Designer.
- Appoint a Principal Contractor.
- Ensure that those that you appoint are competent and adequately resourced to carry out their health and safety duties.
- Ensure that the Principal Contractor has prepared a suitable Construction Phase Plan before the construction work starts.
- Ensure that the project Health and Safety File given to you at the end of the project is kept available for use.

The CDM Regulations 2015 make it clear that the Designer, being one of the first to be appointed and being aware of the Regulations' requirements, must ensure that the Client is alerted to their responsibilities. That is the purpose of this letter.

Please would you reply in acknowledgement that you have received, read and understood this letter. If your response is not received within 10 working days from the date at the top of this letter, the above will be taken as acknowledged.

Yours <Designer's signature>

Sometimes it may be necessary to issue a separate confirmation of the appointment. The negotiations over the appointment may drag on through several iterations and so the CDM notifications should not be mixed up with those. If this is the case, an obvious trigger will be needed to ensure this required obligation on the designer (or principal designer) has been discharged.

For projects over the CDM notification threshold, an F10 form needs to be completed and submitted to the HSE.

### Pre-construction information

The principal designer must ensure that health and safety file information is gathered during the pre-construction phase (see page 149: Stage 4). However, there are very few projects where design stops when the project moves to site. It is therefore important to recognise that the CDM responsibilities continue and that the relevant information needs to be collected for the health and safety file, ready for handover at completion. The principal designer may or may not be retained to undertake this latter phase. If the principal designer is not retained, they must pass the health and safety file information to the principal contractor.

Principal designers will have:

– technical knowledge of the construction industry relevant to the project, and
– experience to manage and coordinate the pre-construction phase and any design work after construction begins.

Principal designers are required to:

– plan, manage, monitor and coordinate health and safety during the pre-construction phase
– ensure the project team works to reduce risks, coordinate information and generate solutions for construction, maintenance and cleaning that are as risk fee and obvious as possible
– generate and organise information for the health and safety file and hand this over at the end of their commission
– organise and ensure circulation of all pre-existing information on the project, and
– ensure that coherent pre-construction information regarding the project – both prior to the current work and as generated by the team – is handed over to the principal contractor.

| Project role | 0 ⟳ Strategic Definition | 1 ⟳ Preparation and Brief | 2 ⟳ Concept Design |
|---|---|---|---|
| Principal contract operations for a design and build project | Client determining procurement contract route | Client appointment of employer's team | Employer's team develop design and Employer's Requirements |
| Principal designer (PD) | Possible appointment | Define appointment under design and build contract | PD undertakes role as in other contracts |
| Principal contractor (PC) | | Possible appointment Liaise with PD | May have early appointment Liaise with existing PD |
| Options: PD client side then switched to contractor | | | |
| PD role undertaken by several bodies | | | |
| PD changes employment; client then contractor | | | |

Figure 1.3   *The principal designer and principal contractor roles on a design and build project*

## The principal contractor

On projects where there will be more than one contractor, the CDM regulations require that one of them be appointed as the principal contractor. Early engagement with the principal contractor is always recommended, although this is not always possible. It can help the design team to determine the best approach to be adopted in the design stages,

| **3** ○ | **4** ○ | **5** ○ | **6** ○ |
|---|---|---|---|
| **Developed Design** | **Technical Design** | **Construction** | **Handover and Close Out** |
| Design requirements identified<br><br>Documents finalised<br><br>Contract tendered/awarded | Contractor appointed<br><br>Team novated or switched. Contractor's Proposals take over from Employer's Requirements | Contractor in authority over complete project | Contractor team hands back to client |
| PD role may finish when PC is appointed | PD role could continue if novated to PC | PD role as part of PC team | PD role completes |
| Determine if PC will take on PD role or existing PD will be novated or new PD appointed to take on role | PD role will continue collecting information from the contractor team | As Stage 4 but ensuring that all design during construction is taken account of and reviewed and information for the H&S file and 'As-constructed' Information is kept up to date | PD as part of PC team contributes to handover and ensures H&S file and 'As-constructed' Information are handed over |

and can allow the principal contractor to propose solutions to complex design issues at an early stage.

Often, while a project is on site, especially under design and build or management contract forms, the authority over any design work is vested with the principal contractor (see figure 1.3) and therefore it is logical that they become the controlling entity during this phase. For traditional and minor works contract forms, authority will remain with the senior designers and clearly the principal designer role is best retained by them in these situations. The principal contractor is now a well-established role, and for most of the industry their responsibilities are clearly understood.

## Assembling the project team

At the end of Stage 1 and before the commencement of Stage 2 the Initial Project Brief should be clear. Its development will help determine the size of the project team, how the roles and responsibilities should be allocated, and what experience is required among the team members.

### Building a project team

At this stage the project team members are likely to be new to each other. Across the industry, it is usual for teams to be formed for specific projects then broken up afterwards. While experienced individuals may work together again over time, this is by far the exception rather than the rule. Therefore, at the early stages of a new project, there is always an element of team members getting used to working with each other. Experienced project managers and other leaders recognise the need to build a team 'spirit'; this can take a while, but it is important for the success of the project that the team gets off to a good start.

There should be some form of induction for new team members as they are appointed, so that everyone will be aware of the project formalities. Informal team-building initiatives can also be highly beneficial from a health and safety perspective. Sometimes, team members are reluctant to discuss or raise issues, so making personal connections often helps in this respect.

### The health and safety adviser

Over recent decades, consultant teams have become larger as the construction industry has become more complex. It is very difficult for a small number of consultants, no matter how skilled, to cover all the subjects needed. Therefore, for some projects the use of a health and safety adviser is a logical option. Indeed, on some large projects whole teams have been devoted to the management of health and safety.

Accumulated good practice experience and feedback from exemplar projects would suggest that this makes sense, certainly for larger projects.

The CDM regulations do not preclude a route for incorporating a health and safety adviser into the project team. Several sectors of the industry have already begun to offer such a service. The challenge will be to ensure that such a person can bring value and support the team's work. The health and safety specialist needs a balance of skills, across design, procurement, negotiation, technical, contracts and finance. They need to see the other professionals' perspectives and be able to help design solutions.

The health and safety adviser must be able to focus on the Project Outcomes, and not get bogged down in process. The CDM regulations, together with a new resolve to join up the industry and greater use of new technologies, such as Building Information Modelling (BIM), will help, supported, of course, by the RIBA Plan of Work 2013. The emergence of a health and safety specialist with the right blend of skills and an approach to suit will be a huge step forward and is to be welcomed. However, they are not the principal designer.

## Schedules of Services

In developing the Schedules of Services, the project team need to be clear about who will undertake what in respect of health and safety. The various responsibilities need to be referenced specifically and the client needs to ensure there are no gaps or overlaps. The structure of the RIBA Plan of Work helps considerably – it can be used to structure the detail of the team members' services around outputs.

Project team members need to review carefully and discuss with the client their Schedule of Services. Often the pressure to make progress with the project will overtake resolution of the fine detail. A well-structured document control process must record and manage the flow of these negotiations. Often they can cover quite a period of time and so some of the exact detail can get lost. Make sure this does not happen and, if necessary, revisit the conclusion so that everyone is clear about what has ultimately been agreed. Avoid using a base document with references to a number of email chains, which are difficult to track and can lead to vague conclusions.

## Design Responsibility Matrix

It is essential that a Design Responsibility Matrix is prepared at this stage. It takes the Schedules of Services to the next level of detail, making clear what the design team members have all agreed individually with the client. The Schedules of Services should specify which health and safety actions each team member will undertake and at what stages or by which milestones they need to be completed. It is essential that the Design Responsibility Matrix is agreed as part of the agreement of professional services contracts. It should be a standard agenda item at every team meeting.

The preparation of the Design Responsibility Matrix often leads to tasks and responsibilities that have not been allocated to team members being identified. Health and safety issues are often among such loose ends.

It is likely that not all the design team members will be on board at this stage; the matrix should therefore also identify future appointments and their areas of responsibility.

It is also essential that the matrix identifies primary and supporting roles. It may be necessary for more than one team member to contribute to a particular activity; in such instances, the matrix should make clear who has managerial authority.

### Contractual Tree

The Contractual Tree is a document aligned with the Schedules of Services and the Design Responsibilities Matrix. It identifies the contractual

### CDM responsibilities

Authorities such as the HSE often find it difficult to identify who is in authority on a particular project. As the CDM regulations place core responsibilities on the client and the principal designer, the contractual authority of each party should match their statutory responsibilities, if at all possible.

There have been instances where infringements concerning scaffolding have resulted in the HSE visiting the architects' offices. After often lengthy and embarrassing questioning, the inspectors were convinced that, contractually, the designers had no authority or ability to influence the scaffolding operations.

Including the contractual relationships in a straightforward document, as part of the project essentials, will help to prevent such misunderstandings arising.

relationships between the project team members. It can also be used to clarify their responsibilities, as there is often confusion over who has authority, especially where there is involvement by agencies outside the team. This document helps to ensure that the team members themselves understand the various relationships, so that a consistent approach will be adopted.

## Drafting project documents

Always consider how a person new to the project would understand a document. To be effective, each document has to read as a stand-alone piece of information.

### Technology and Communication Strategies

The Project Strategies covering how technology will be used and communication conducted on the project need to be clearly established.

A number of different core technologies are available for running projects. The choice of technology will determine which software should be used across the project. Equally, the hardware selected for recording or reproducing information must be able to fully support the processes.

Software standards change rapidly. As a result, software is increasingly aiding design and information manipulation. This can be used to ensure all designs have properly considered the health and safety issues, and that these can be recorded separately and identified, eg visually in matrix form.

## Reality check

Software can sometimes lead designers into a false sense of security – perhaps leading them to claim something is resolved when it is not. A reality check is always worthwhile, if possible undertaken by someone outside the team.

### CIC BIM Protocol

The Construction Industry Council (CIC) *BIM Protocol* requires that software and communications standards are established during Stage 0, which can be expanded at this stage as more project details become available.

The CIC *BIM Protocol* can be downloaded from http://cic.org.uk/publications

Whatever systems are used, agreed communication channels must be implemented at this time, so that issues can be shared with the whole design team and, if necessary, the client, and comments quickly assembled. This makes finding a rounded, objective solution much more straightforward.

The media and methods to be used on the project need to be agreed across the team. These may range from the setting up of a project website or an intranet to the use of the PDF file format for all project

### Client protocols

The protocols used by clients can sometimes hinder communications. The resulting potential for misunderstandings will create unnecessary project risks.

On a large project with a well-established client, the client demanded that the whole team use a particular project intranet. The system brought in and paid for by the client was advertised for large projects and contained many attributes to the client's liking. However, all of these were from the client's perspective. From the average team member's position, working on the system was time intensive, viewing other members' work was difficult and finding exactly what other information was available was very problematic.

Very quickly the team developed their own 'method' of transmitting information (as PDFs), circumventing the intranet. Information uploaded to the intranet was deemed 'just for the client'.

documents. However, the methods adopted need to be in proportion to the project, and straightforward for all members of the team to use. Do not let the medium overtake the essence of simple, practical exchange of information.

A project intranet that is owned and effectively controlled by the client, or perhaps the principal contractor, can be turned off at any stage. It is therefore not recommend that the Health and Safety Strategy or the background information relating to health and safety decisions is only held on the intranet. A separate record of these issues needs to be kept on secure storage in the originator's office. This is also useful for reference purposes and for ensuring that the health and safety file includes all the necessary information.

## Health and safety on small projects

On a small project there are limited resources, therefore time and experience might simply not be as available as on a larger project. This can affect the application of health and safety practices. To the HSE, small projects are a critical area of interest as they account for a disproportionate number of the accidents that occur on construction sites. On a small project, there needs to be an emphasis on using simple, straightforward and clear processes. These must focus on the essentials:

– Establish the key principles early on.
– Identify the critical participants.
– Explain the responsibilities to the client (see page 55) and get confirmation of their understanding in writing.
– The essential principles can still be followed, but should be adapted to suit the size of the project. Use the same templates, but with fewer options.
– Do as much as possible visually.
– Keep everything as simple as possible.
– Use third party references, especially HSE documents, as much as possible.
– Get everyone focused on designing out risk.
– Motivate everyone to work safely.
– Make it a matter of pride, not an issue of threat or blame.

## Site Information

The provision of Site Information, both legally and logically, is the responsibility of the client. On larger projects this information is gathered by specialist surveyors, on behalf of the client, as they can assemble accurate detail relatively quickly. The client may engage the surveyor directly, or this might be part of the design team's responsibilities. Whoever undertakes the survey work, it should be made very clear by the client, or the client's representative, that all surveying is to be undertaken safely and with minimal risk to those going on site.

Surveyors should be given access to whatever information already exists. This might not be reliable, but it will at least provide a starting point, and it may throw up clues as to the nature of the site. Experienced surveyors can read any signs in existing information that will alert them to possible dangers and problems.

Those going on site must be aware of physical hazards, such as wells or hidden shafts, unstable structures and, of course, the presence of asbestos and other toxins. There may also be hazards from animals and, if the site has been used by vagrants, from discarded needles or drugs.

There are some general rules for going on site at the commencement of the project:

I Assemble all information available, and make an assessment of possible hazards.
I Ensure those going on site have the necessary experience and training.
I Go well equipped, with copies of the existing information, correct protective clothing and equipment, mobile phones, camera and appropriate weather protection.
I Always let the office know your plans and when you expect to return.
I Never take risks, especially entering abandoned buildings – they often have unsafe structures and services or have infestations.
I If any unseen problems occur, the visit must be called off.

### Feasibility Studies

At Stage 1, it is possible that several sites will have to be appraised before one can be chosen – the health and safety information needs to be part of the decision-making process.

It is likely that a number of critical issues will be flagged up during this process, although sometimes these will remain unknown until a detailed exploration has been undertaken. It is important to ensure that all the potential factors are examined and that all findings are reported to the client and the design team.

While the site arrangement for the building is yet to be fixed, the design team should consider any difficulties arising from potential layouts that could be hazardous. Often other parameters, such as planning consent, fire regulations and good design criteria, mean that sites must have a reasonable layout. However, surrounding traffic and road layouts outside the site, topography and geology can conspire to create difficult situations. The design team need to bring these into their thinking and, when the layout is finalised, develop guidance for the construction team.

### Health and safety considerations

It is essential that the design team start with as clear a picture as possible. Any Site Information must be considered from the perspective of health and safety implications, so that it can be fed into any Feasibility Studies and the developing Initial Project Brief. Do not make assumptions that a particular site is safe or that, because there are no obvious indicators of potential issues, everything is alright – some difficult problems might lie just below the surface.

Issues such as asbestos, unsafe services, hidden structural defects or underground cavities need to be identified as early as possible as the costs of remedial measures might make the site unviable. In extreme

### Site investigation

A project was at an early stage when the detailed site analysis identified that gas holders which were thought to be disused were in fact still live. As they were too close to the proposed dwellings, the project had to be put on hold until the gas holders were no longer in use.

circumstances, health and safety issues not identified during the site investigations can result in work on site being stopped.

Copies of any asbestos registers or documents confirming the locations of structures or safety measures undertaken previously need to be included in the information available.

### Site approach and surroundings

Site Information should include some details of the area outside the site, so that wider health and safety issues can be identified. For example, the transport systems adjacent to the site – the roads in particular – need to be reviewed. Will construction traffic cause congestion? Will the complex vehicle movements cause problems? Can traffic flow and pedestrians be segregated? Are there bottlenecks that can be eased? Are there nearby schools, hospitals, superstores, transport interchanges or other high-volume traffic centres? Thought also needs to be given to how traffic will be managed once work has started on site.

Significant pipelines, cables and drainage, even pending roadworks, should also be considered.

From this analysis, the best site access, both temporary and permanent, can be judged. Time considerations for deliveries, movements of large plant and control of contaminants may need to be factored in – these are often overlooked by the design team.

Make a clear proposal based on these issues, either within or as a supplement to any Feasibility Study for the client. Ensure these are flagged up for later discussion with the contractor, once they are appointed.

### On-site features

Most design teams will want to make the most of any on-site features, such as changes in level, watercourses or geological features. There are, however, many characteristics of the site that could be hazardous if not considered early on and factored into the project. Rivers, streams, lakes and low-lying areas can all bring significant risks that need to be considered. In recent decades, problems due to weather-related events (eg flooding and mud slides) have become more common.

## Surveys for small projects

Specialist surveyors are rarely employed on small projects – it is likely that the site analysis will be undertaken by one of the design team. It is essential that whoever undertakes the survey takes safety seriously, by applying all the principles of site safety and taking all necessary precautions. It may seem disproportionate for a small project, but even on the smallest of sites, hazards lurk for the unwary.

– Hidden and disused wells that are not on any records are common on small sites.
– Disused buildings may have infestations of wild animals – even pigeons represent a significant health hazard, as breathing in particles from their droppings is dangerous, and Weil's disease can be contracted from watercourses inhabited by rats.

Always ensure you go to site well prepared, and if you have to go alone, make sure the office and others know your plans and when to expect you to return.

Design teams need to be alive to these issues and ensure they have correctly accounted for them, as a direct obligation under the CDM regulations.

### Terrain and surface details

The general principles described in Stage 0 can now start to be applied to the specific details of the project. Identifying these at this stage will help with design development later. Making best use of the terrain will bring its own challenges. In looking at the surface levels and the project requirements, designers need to be aware of the features that they may be required to address to achieve the Project Objectives.

Using the natural gradient of the site is a common design feature. It is important to ensure that any subsequent design can work with the fall, not against it. A need for deep excavations or basement levels will immediately raise the level of hazard, and there must be enough space to undertake excavation safely.

On a cramped or complex site, eg with several underground issues, the tendering and design specifications need to allow for a higher degree of expertise than would be required for a simpler situation. Now is the time for such issues to be identified and made known to the client, so that the time and cost implications can be factored into the overall budget and programme.

## Existing structures and services

There are likely to be existing hazards above and below any site that will have to be worked around or removed. Across the site there may be electrical cables, sewers, culverts, open drains, tunnels or pipelines.

Existing structures, whether above or below ground, have a built-in potential to cause harm, even for the team surveying the site. These need to be examined in detail as early as possible to ensure there is a comprehensive understanding of their condition.

Whether the existing structures are being built into the new works or removed, they will need to be controlled. It is the responsibility of the designers to understand how this is to be done and to offer the construction team a viable solution.

Services installations can also be extremely hazardous. Once the site is known, detailed desk-top and on-site examinations need to be undertaken, especially for urban sites or where there is known to be a high density of services.

It is common for sites to contain services that have not been recorded. Therefore, for sites that are suspected to have been 'well used' in the past, any exploratory work that can be done will be beneficial. This is good health and safety practice and often pays dividends by minimising delays.

## Retained structures

Retained structures must be treated with equal care, the potentially difficult areas being structural integrity, asbestos content and hidden services. These all need to be identified. As with underground issues, the design team will have to identify how the risks are going to be controlled. This may involve complex temporary works for structural considerations, bunding or more extensive preparations.

### Contamination

It is common for sites have some form of contamination and so this needs to be factored into any site review.

## Project Execution Plan

The development of the Project Execution Plan is essential for the appropriate governance of the project. It pulls together all the key overarching elements of the client's requirements and desired outcomes. It should be the reference that everyone goes back to, ensuring that the project is on course. A continuous element of the plan is health and safety.

From Stage 1, the health and safety focus of the Project Execution Plan should be clearly seen in the day-to-day working of the project. All the design considerations, the analysis, the planning and development will have this focus – not specifically drawn out, but as a matter of everyday working.

The focus on health and safety should not be something of special note, but part of the normal project considerations – always there but not singled out. This is sometimes looked upon as something of a challenge, but setting up the right processes and systems at the start makes this less so. Creating the right atmosphere is the key.

## Handover Strategy

The Handover Strategy for a building should include all the requirements for phased handovers, commissioning, training of staff and any other factors crucial to the successful occupation of the building. On some projects, the Building Services Research and Information Association (BSRIA) Soft Landings process is used as the basis for formulating the strategy and for any Post-occupancy Evaluation. The Government Soft Landings methodology has also been developed for use on BIM projects (see page 190: Stage 6).

Early stage consultations, surveys or monitoring may be undertaken as necessary to establish sustainability criteria or assessment procedures.

## Risk assessments

Risk assessment is a fundamental activity for health and safety, but it should not be confused with the wider project Risk Assessment process.

### Project Risk Assessment

This subject is covered in more detail in the *RIBA Plan of Work 2013 Guide: Design Management.*

Health and safety risk assessments have had a chequered history. Frequently they are not used, and are consigned to be a piece of dead paperwork sitting on a shelf and of no real tangible benefit.

Risk assessments should only be used where they will have an impact on the workplace or the manner in which any tasks are undertaken, improving what otherwise would be a hazardous undertaking. Pressuring the team to produce assessments that are not used is unhelpful and wastes resources. This approach needs to be resisted, and good practice alternatives applied instead.

Various methods of risk assessment can be used. However, the numerical matrix is to be avoided. This method entails assigning numerical values for both harm and risk to the various elements of the project, which are then consolidated to arrive at a number representing the overall level of risk. Some parts of the industry continue to use this method, but it is a disconnected, opinion-based approach that has very little relevance in practice.

It is better to approach risk assessment by asking: What do we need to do to achieve safety? How do we deliver that message, clearly and simply?

More often than not, this means adopting simple measures, with clear logic, no complex language and, preferably, using almost entirely visual means. As the consultant team are well versed in generating and reviewing drawings, it is therefore sensible to use drawings and visual methods to identify risk areas and issues. The 'visual risk matrix' is one of the standout methods for doing this. It comprises a simple matrix identifying all potential issues but using a visual representation. This may not always be possible, but using a mixture of simple messages and visual means can be nearly as effective. The red–amber–green list (RAG list) is a simple but effective alternative.

At this stage, it is essential that the approach to be adopted by the team is made clear, and that everyone has signed up to it. In this way, messages from different parts of the team can be linked together and be much more powerful.

### Health and safety initiatives

Since the Construction Safety Summit of 2001, many industry initiatives have come to prominence. Some have been the source of good practice and continue to deliver worthwhile guidance.

Of note currently are:

- Proportionate and Practicable – an RIBA initiative
- CDM Differently and Safety Visually – a CIC initiative
- Breathe Freely – a Land Securities sponsored initiative.

## Information Exchanges

Information Exchanges required for Stage 1 are as follows:

| at stage completion: the Initial Project Brief
| for UK Government projects: an output of Project Information is required.

At this stage the amount of information exchanged, principally in the form of the Initial Project Brief, will start to increase. The Information Exchanges need to be organised, so that the team are guided by a well-structured method, with health and safety information always being included. Building good practice into the project at this stage saves time and effort later on.

This methodology needs to identify the 'how', 'when' and 'what', and include the structure that all information should be based on. This should also state how health and safety information will be included and how it will be identified, described and processed (see 'Risk assessments', above).

Good quality Information Exchanges are as much about setting up and following a well-structured, robust system as they are about ensuring good communication. Setting this out as a published set of rules and process maps may seem excessive, but it establishes clarity and expectations. These make for easy, efficient and reliable Information Exchanges.

### Document mark up

In the design development stages, where drawings are circulated between the team, marking up documents with health and safety issues provides a simple and very clear method of identifying issues or progress in resolving them. The use of electronic or hand-applied notes and tags leaves a record in the Project Information and helps others in the team see the issues. While this approach is normally used for design development, it is highly effective at resolving health and safety issues. It is a good idea to ensure that the procedures established at this stage allow for this system to be implemented.

## Chapter summary 1

This is the stage that really sets the scene for the project. Developing a rapport with the client and making sure there is a commitment to health and safety is essential.

Getting off to a good start always requires preparation and hard work. This will pay dividends later on, as the project expands and becomes more complex. The underlying objectives and principles embedded in the project will provide a structure, and ensure everything stays on course.

Making sure the right team structure, briefings and procedures are in place is part of the essence of this stage. If the whole team are clear about these from this point on, it will be much easier to ensure they continue to be applied consistently until the very end.

All approaches must fit the project. The approach to health and safety must be in proportion and relevant to the size, complexity and procurement route. It is definitely not the case that one size fits all.

Key issues to consider at this stage include the following:

| Details of the Initial Project Brief must be in place.
| The health and safety aspirations need to be in place and signed off by the client and the team.
| All roles and responsibilities need to be close to identification.
| Communication procedures and team structure should be agreed.
| Feasibility Studies must place a strong emphasis on safe working and identify any health and safety issues.
| Details of processes going forward should be planned in draft.
| Everyone needs to have a clear idea of how the overall health and safety approach is going to be applied.

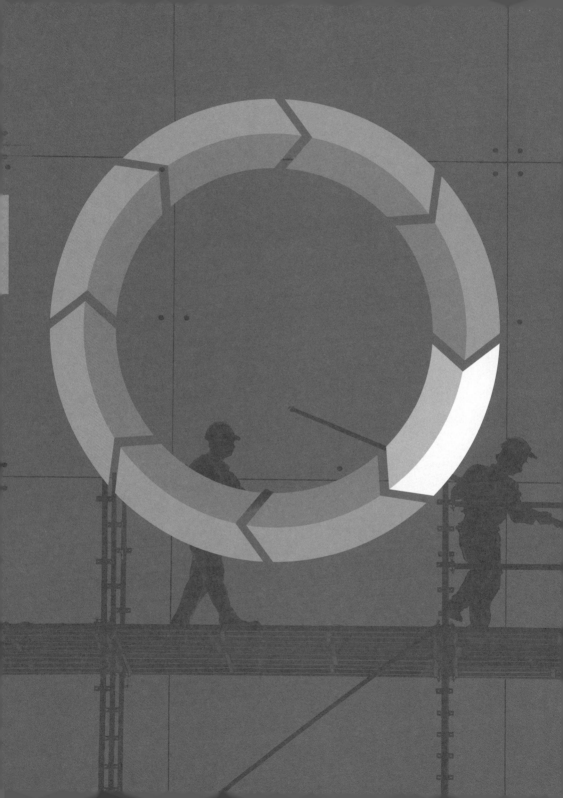

# Stage 2

# Concept Design

# Chapter overview

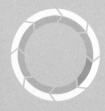

The Concept Design stage starts with an assimilation of the information gathered to date, principally the Site Information, the Feasibility Studies and the Initial Project Brief.

The Construction Strategy is an important reference point, framing the key issues across the project as a whole. The development of the Health and Safety Strategy should always bear in mind the construction implications.

It is important that, whatever the project, it has an underlying intellectual framework – a cohesiveness that binds the individual thoughts together to achieve a comprehensible approach. That framework should encompass a consideration of health and safety. As a result, the early ideas will be developed in a way that considers the risks to those involved in the construction, use or maintenance of the building.

During Stage 2, the Concept Design will be developed iteratively, in response to the Initial Project Brief and in line with comments from the client, other stakeholders and the design team.

The principles identified in the previous stages should start to be applied to particular elements of the project. Health and safety in itself should be part of the decision-making approaches directing the design, not just a means to an end. It is a part, not a whole – an influencing guiding element. It always needs to be part of the decision-making process but should not dominate it.

All of these elements use the processes that were set in motion in previous stages. It should also be plain that health and safety analysis, while important, should not be pursued to the exclusion of all else: it must not assume an all-pervading importance, it must be in proportion.

Stage 2 is about the realisation of the initial ideas, and ensuring that the outcomes that emerge will be ready for the developed technical design work in Stage 3.

Stage 2 also continues the framework of good governance, the structure of the administration, the process of realistic assessment and managing the design. The design team must continue to focus on and give careful consideration to analysis of risk across the project design.

**The key coverage in this chapter is as follows:**

The Health and Safety Strategy

CDM considerations at Stage 2

The health and safety information sets

The balance of risk and design

Concept Design and health and safety

Opportunities and risks

Finalising the Concept Design

Information Exchanges

# Introduction

Creating a Concept Design is all about balancing the possible with the achievable. It is the stage when the Project Objectives are translated into tangible deliverables, in the form of exchanged information that reflects the Initial Project Brief. The design team need to take account of any ongoing issues and craft a Concept Design that can be agreed with the client.

This stage will involve considering many options and narrowing them down relatively quickly. The project needs to progress sufficiently to enable planning applications and other necessary formal activities to be commenced. There may also be testing of ideas, to ensure that they are capable of being developed in the later technical design stages.

*From Stage 1*
It is important to take full advantage of the Stage 1 preparations.

Ensure the health and safety aspirations are in place and being applied.

Ensure the client understands their responsibilities.

Project procedures covering health and safety should be in place.

Team working should include health and safety measures.

The approach to site health and safety issues will be becoming clear.

The possible health and safety issues related to the contract and procurement route must be clearly understood.

## What are the Core Objectives of this stage?

The Core Objectives of the RIBA Plan of Work 2013 at Stage 2 are:

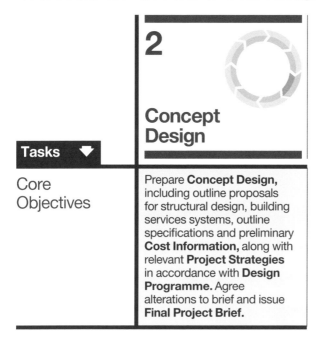

The Core Objectives at this stage revolve around the development of the Concept Design and constantly referencing and adjusting the brief until it is aligned to the final Concept Design as the Final Project Brief. At the start of this stage, a number of ideas for the Concept Design need to be tested sufficiently to ensure that the range of possible options is quickly narrowed. The initial and strategic designs for structures and services and the environmental considerations all need to be developed in parallel, reviewed by the lead designer. This will give a clear indication of whether the design is on track and the health and safety elements are under control.

For this stage to be concluded successfully, it is essential that the client and design team foster good working relationships and work collaboratively. These early relationships within the project team must be balanced and well formulated, as they will set the scene for the project as a whole.

## The Health and Safety Strategy

The principles that were set out in the health and safety aspirations now need to be revisited, and reviewed against the emerging design. A vast number of tasks must be carried out, but their exact timing will vary depending on the character of the project. Smaller projects are relatively straightforward. For very large projects, the engagement of a health and safety adviser offers good value because the level of complexity and interactions involved would otherwise absorb resources from others in the team.

### The strategy

Lifting health and safety to an exemplar level is good business practice. To achieve this, it is important that the strategy for dealing with health and safety is thoroughly embedded at this point. Key messages that need to be emphasised throughout the early stages include the following:

I Health and safety is a top agenda item.
I Health and safety issues are the concern of everyone in the team.
I Every issue counts, no matter how small.
I View each situation from everyone's perspective.
I Treat health like safety.
I Information and cooperation are critical – never stop attempting to get the best.

### Developers raising the bar

Several significant UK-based property clients have enhanced requirements for all members of their supply chain. They believe that leadership comes from the client. In order to be appointed, a company must demonstrate a commitment to health and safety beyond that required by regulation and a track record that identifies delivered results. This also includes regular assessments and in-house training from the client over expected performance, which starts with the bullet points listed above.

The box on pages 85–86 gives examples of how these key messages can be incorporated into the strategy.

Once the strategy has been fully developed it needs to be communicated to and implemented by everyone on the project team, including the most senior management. Subsequently, it can be developed and enhanced, and it must be explained to all those who join in later stages.

A key approach is to make sure that the client and other members of the team are well aware of their responsibilities, and that the Health and Safety Strategy continues to remain intact and provide a constant reference across the project. This is covered in detail later.

### Health and Safety Strategy examples

#### Health and safety is a top agenda item
– Every meeting, agenda and report starts with health and safety.
– The client issues a statement to everyone working on the project outlining their support for health and safety.
– Audits and feedback are given to the client on a regular basis to ensure the top agenda commitment is maintained.

#### Health and safety issues are the concern of everyone in the team
– Open communications from everyone on the project. Anyone can raise any issue at any time (supported by a confidential email system that allows anonymous reporting).
– Regular discussions between workers, unions and employers, to discuss health and safety performance.

#### Every issue counts, no matter how small
– Everyone is encouraged to discuss even the smallest issues. Improvements can be made through just the tiniest incremental changes – real progress can be made through hundreds of small improvements.

#### View each situation from everyone's perspective
– Everyone on the project sees it from a different angle and there is often an untapped value in these different views. Everyone is encouraged to speak from their own perspective, not from a prepared approach.

#### Treat health like safety
– Great efforts have been made to reduce physical risks – in reality this has been about safety. An equal focus on health matters is now needed as too many workers suffer from

### Health and Safety Strategy examples (*continued*)

construction-related health issues. The challenge is that most of these effects are very long term. Improving awareness of these effects can and has made a real difference.

**Information and cooperation are critical – never stop attempting to get the best**

- Continually rework communications to improve the understanding that is achieved. There is always a better way to explain – drawn and visual communication has been shown to work best, as it has no language barriers. Much of the industry already uses this as the main form of communication.
- With better communication comes greater empathy and this achieves greater cooperation. A team willing to fully cooperate is a team that will look after each other's interests and is ultimately safer.

## The variable task bars

The key tasks at this stage all require a degree of health and safety focus. Ensuring this is part of the project culture is critical. The RIBA Plan of Work 2013's variable task bars – which cover procurement, programme and (town) planning – can help to achieve the client's various project requirements.

### Procurement

The choice of procurement route for the project can have health and safety implications. The RIBA Plan of Work 2013 is suitable for a range of routes, including traditional, design and build and management forms of contracting. These are covered in more detail in Stage 1 (page 48).

### Programme

The Project Programme also has an impact on health and safety. Sufficient time is needed to ensure that adequate management and resources are dedicated to all operations. It is a requirement of CDM that the client ensures adequate resources, including time, are allowed to undertake the project safely. If too little time is allowed or the programme is excessively optimistic it will lead to increased risk.

## Planning

Planning application development and discussions should be undertaken as the design emerges (figure 2.1). Initially, this will be about the options that are available. It is likely to be about the local authority's attitude and the local plan. It is essential that the site issues previously outlined in detail are monitored during the formulation of the town planning application details.

### Procurement route and Concept Design

The procurement route needs to be considered during the development of the Concept Design, if not earlier. To ensure that risk is properly managed throughout the project, the principles enshrined in the information need to be correctly and clearly communicated. The various procurement routes place authority in different hands, so a change to the route can result in important health and safety decisions being lost.

Ensuring there is clarity on what needs to be communicated and its implications makes this less of a problem. At Stage 2, ensure this is framed clearly as the Concept Design is developed – it will become more important during the next stages.

## CDM considerations at Stage 2

The CDM activities at this stage centre on the need to coordinate the work of the various designers, particularly in relation to the health and safety aspects of the developing design.

If the project requires the appointment of a principal designer, this is likely to have been completed during Stage 1. Under the CDM regulations, the principal designer will have control over the pre-construction phase. They are responsible for ensuring that, so far as is reasonably practicable, any foreseeable risks to the health and safety of people likely to be affected by the project are eliminated or controlled.

The CDM regulations also require that certain documents are prepared during the pre-construction phase, for use during the Construction and In Use stages (see below, page 90).

| | **0** Strategic Definition | **1** Preparation and Brief |
|---|---|---|
| Client | Develop Business Case<br>Review range of sites<br>Commission Feasibility Studies and site surveys<br>Look at options for planning strategy<br>Consider what team members and specialists are needed | Complete Initial Project Brief<br>Finish Feasibility Studies and review of sites<br>Complete strategy<br>Appoint team for early stage work |
| Planning specialist (may be planner, architect, designer or other) | Appointment and review of scope of services<br>May take on role of principal designer (PD) or a separate PD may be appointed<br>If no appointment, default is that PD role lies with designer<br>PD should make position clear in writing | Review sites with the client and develop the Initial Project Brief<br>Actions needed under CDM<br>Review Feasibility Studies and ensure risks are reviewed<br>Start information for the H&S file and pre-construction phase information<br>Start to identify planning constraints |
| Planning specialist (taking on principal designer role) | Note: PD role defaults to designer if no arrangement is made<br>Arrange separate appointment for PD role<br>Agree Schedule of Services<br>Make sure the client is aware of their CDM duties and what the PD will do<br>Start to assist collation of information on sites, strategy and possible team expertise<br>Possible start of H&S file and pre-construction phase information | Ensure the client is aware of roles<br>Assist with form F10 submission if applicable<br>Develop information on chosen site<br>Develop/start information for the H&S file and pre-construction information<br>As and when team appointed, encourage cooperation and coordination of H&S issues |
| Planning preparation<br>Planning application made | ← | ← |

Figure 2.1 Town planning and the principal designer

| **2** <br> **Concept** <br> **Design** | **3** <br> **Developed** <br> **Design** |
|---|---|
| Review sites or agree site details with project team <br><br> Ensure strategy in place <br><br> Ensure H&S Strategy and requirements in place | If team members are changing, ensure there is a full handover between members <br><br> Ensure Schedules of Services for outgoing and incoming teams match |
| Develop the design with others if necessary <br><br> Identify planning application details <br><br> Possible town planning application made <br><br> Ensure H&S issues have been identified and reviewed <br><br> Massing, layout, materials and cleanability need lowest risk options to be identified | Possible town planning application made <br><br> Processes as Stage 2 but in more detail <br><br> As detail increases, keep information reviewed and updated <br><br> If role is to finish, ensure that actions undertaken are clearly recorded |
| Actions are as Stage 2 plus develop team working and information gathering <br><br> Ensure that as detail increases, risk analysis continues and risks are minimised <br><br> Record key decisions | Actions are as Stage 2 plus, if role is to end, ensure there is a comprehensive and detailed handover to those taking on the PD role <br><br> May be necessary to brief others depending on the complexity of the project |

## The health and safety information sets

Among the obligations of the principal designer is the assembly and organisation of relevant information (figure 2.2). There are two aspects to this. The first is the assembly of all information about the project and the site before design development gets under way. The second is the development of the health and safety pre-construction information. This will contain all the elements of the design, and ensure the construction team are aware of them. It will then be developed to include construction information and eventually be handed over to the client at handover as an operations manual. In a BIM-enabled project, this will all be achieved with data transfers.

### Pre-construction information

A lot of information needs to have been collected or produced before the design phase can commence. All relevant information needs to be known about the site, including its locality, the status of any existing structures and the town planning situation.

All of this information must be pulled together and shared across the project team. As the client may not appoint all of the project team members together, it is particularly important that any new project team members have access to exactly the same information. The various design team members will also have a range of perspectives. Providing everyone with all the information that is available is a significant step towards good health and safety practice, ensuring a common starting point.

To summarise, the information needed at the start of Stage 2 includes:

I Initial Project Brief, including the Project Objectives
I Project Execution Plan
I all Site Information, including:
  o physical and environmental conditions
  o existing structures
  o detailed location information
  o surrounding infrastructure
  o topography
  o geology
  o climate, etc

**Start of project**

**Client** to check what documents are already in their possession that will be relevant to the project, eg an existing health and safety file.

**Pre-construction information (PCI)**

**Client and principal designer (PD)** must work together to:

– assess adequacy of existing information (eg existing health and safety file from earlier project or asbestos survey)

– agree arrangements to fill gaps in existing information

– provide sufficient information to designers and contractors.

**Process of design**

**Designers** must take account of PCI to:

– eliminate, reduce or control foreseeable risks in their designs, and

– provide information to the PD about measures taken in designs to reduce or control risks not eliminated.

**PD** to use this information to:

– take it into account in the PCI and the health and safety file, and

– provide it to the principal contractor (PC) towards the construction phase plan.

**Construction phase plan**

– **Client** to ensure the plan is drawn up before construction phase begins.

– **PC** to draw up the plan on the basis of:

– pre-construction information, and

– information provided with designs.

**PD** to help the PC prepare the plan.

**PC** to:

– ensure the plan is appropriately reviewed, updated and revised

– address any significant changes to risks involved and controls put in place.

**Health and safety file**

– **Client** to ensure the PD prepares the file.

– **PD** to prepare the file in cooperation with the PC.

– **PD** to ensure the file is appropriately updated, reviewed and revised.

– **PC** to provide PD with relevant information for inclusion in the file.

– **PD** to pass the file to the client at the end of the project.

– **PD** to pass the file to the PC if the PD's appointment ends before the project finishes.

**End of project**

– **Client** to retain the health and safety file and ensure it is available for any subsequent construction work on the building.

– If the **client** disposes of their interest in the building, they must provide the file to anyone who takes on the client duties.

**Note:** This diagram shows how the various types of information relate to each other and influence the content of other types of information during the construction process (the arrows show the possible different flows of information). So, for example as pre-construction information is developed, this influences the risks designers should consider and the information they provide about how their designs reduce or control foreseeable risks. In turn, this may influence further development of the pre-construction information, as well as the construction phase plan and the health and safety file.

*Figure 2.2   Types of information on a project with more than one contractor*

- town planning history and local plan information, including planning constraints
- Feasibility Studies, current and previously undertaken
- Project Budget
- outline Project Programme
- Project Strategies:
  - Health and Safety Strategy
  - procurement strategy
  - Sustainability Strategy
  - Maintenance and Operational Strategy.

Every one of the above has a health and safety element, which needs to be clearly identified during the design development, taking on board the principles of assessment, review and removal or reduction of any potential risks.

## Design phase CDM information

The CDM regulations require the preparation of two types of specific information:

- The health and safety file – prepared by the principal designer, and containing all information that may be needed to manage the health and safety of the building after it has been handed over. The file will be handed over to the client during Stage 6: Handover and Close Out.
- The construction phase plan – prepared by the principal contractor, with the assistance of the principal designer, and setting out the health and safety arrangements that will apply during the construction phase.

The preparation of the health and safety file will commence at Stage 2, with the development of the Concept Design. Depending on when the contractor is appointed, the construction phase plan may also be started at this stage.

### Health and safety file

The level of detail contained in the health and safety file needs to be in proportion to the size or complexity of the project (see page 149: Stage 4). The file needs to be a useful and practical document, therefore its contents should be clear and relevant – including detail for the sake of it is unhelpful, and blindly copying information into it serves little purpose other than to hinder those who will later rely on this information.

### Construction phase plan

The project design team and contractor must set out the construction sequence and health and safety arrangements for the project so that they are properly understood by all parties involved on site. Taking its lead from the Health and Safety Strategy, the construction phase plan should continue to enforce the headline principles established for the project (see page 147: Stage 4).

### HSE guidance

The HSE has produced a range of *Busy builder* leaflets and a 'CDM Wizard' app, which provide information and guidance for the pre-construction phase.

## The balance of risk and design

Risk is always there in everyday life – it is present in everything we do. Some people in the health and safety world have come to view risk exclusively as a regulatory compliance issue. In their eyes, compliance with the regulations is good, any hint of non-compliance is bad. However, construction design just does not fit into such a simple analysis. The thought that all issues can be covered by mapping out a strict process that ultimately leads to compliance with regulations and a tick in a box is to miss the nuances and complexities within the design process. It focuses too much on the statistics, and not enough on the end result.

### Rethinking safety

A rethink of what this is all about was covered by Andrew Townsend in his book *Safety Can't Be Measured* (Gower, 2013). He looked at how statistics have to some degree controlled the health and safety world, and to no real overall benefit.

No design should be limited by health and safety considerations, but it must take account of them. In taking a design forward, the design team should consider it from all perspectives. That is why a team with a wide spread of experience and knowledge is needed. It is always important to realise that not every eventuality can be allowed for. The construction team and others should also be sufficiently able and experienced to understand commonly used principles and materials.

It may be that to satisfy other issues the contractor will take on a less safe option – this is where experience is needed to control risks to acceptable levels.

## Reducing construction risks

### Think outside the tick box

Often, tick box forms of risk assessment are based on strict compliance with perceived best practice: for example, do not specify or use concrete blocks over 20kg. However, dense blocks can be very effective where a high level of acoustic performance is required. Ignoring the tick box form and instead designing in the use of mechanical handling or off-site manufactured units is potentially a better answer. Often, thinking outside the box is prevented by a concentration on regulatory compliance.

### Understand the real problem

Often an issue may be about behaviour rather than design. Traditionally, full sheets of plasterboard are specified for interior linings. This gives rise to a manual handling issue, as several sheets may have to be offloaded into place by one worker. Specifying half boards has not worked. The real issue for workers is the speed of delivery to the workface, so workers tend to carry more sheets at a time. On large installations, it would be appropriate to consider adopting fully mechanical palletised handling.

### Off-site assembly

Many elements can be preassembled off site, in factory conditions. This avoids the need for cutting and complex operations on site, sometimes in hazardous locations. Elements such as roof perimeters, flues and chimneys, balconies, balustrades, windows, rainwater systems, cladding and many masonry units can benefit from off-site assembly.

## Reducing construction risks (*continued*)

### Project layout

When designing the foundations and underground works of a simple building, the designer must take account of both the site constraints and the needs of the brief. The structural engineer will offer solutions based on structural characteristics, the services engineer will consider where the drains, cables and pipes need to be and, if available, the contractor will identify the most practical construction sequence.

Each will have their own perspective and preferred approach. They need to have an understanding of the risks under their design remit, but also an appreciation of those that lie with the rest of the team. These have to be pulled together to ensure they do not combine to generate increased risk and, if possible, sequenced or designed in such a way as to reduce or eliminate risk. Health and safety will be one consideration among several, but not necessarily the dominant one.

### High-level working

Larger projects often require high-level working, an obvious example being The Shard in London. It is entirely acceptable to control the risks involved, rather than attempt to design them out. The use of rope access can be of great benefit and allows safety and design to be approached in a balanced way. The UK's safety record for rope access when used by skilled professionals is second to none (see irata.org).

### The logic process

One way of undertaking this design approach would be to follow a logic process, such as the following.

## Step 1

Examine each design element by asking the following questions:

I  Question 1
   Is the design commonplace for this size, type and class of project?

| Question 2

Does the design use materials, processes and construction sequences that do not give rise to unnecessary activities (such as cutting on site), and will it be safe in use and to clean and maintain?

If the answers to questions 1 and 2 are both yes, it is not worth bringing the element to the attention of the wider project team.

*Note*: If most of the design is of this category then record this in the health and safety file.

| Question 3

Is the design uncommon for this size, type and class of project? For example:

○ uncommon use of materials (either new materials or unusual use of common ones)
○ uncommon sequences or assembly techniques
○ uncommon requirements for tolerances, quality or timing.

If the answer to question 3 is yes, the design needs further detailed consideration. Can something be changed to take away the uncertainty or the potential to do harm? Often it can, and a good, rounded team approach can help to identify what. However, changing one parameter could give rise to other issues and therefore require a further cycle of consideration.

Eventually this process shakes out everything that reasonably can be expected to be done, while ensuring that the design aspirations are maintained.

**Step 2**

Highlight the remaining items, if any, to the construction team, the client and, if relevant, to whoever will be using and maintaining the building.

**Step 3**

Record all key decisions, but in a proportionate way.

When developing a design, the challenge is to determine how much risk each element is adding to the project. Of course, this is a very taxing question in practice. As to the question how much is too much, that is down to professional judgement and experience.

# Concept Design and health and safety

In undertaking the Concept Design development, it is essential that the design team do not become overly focused on health and safety issues. The CDM regulations and the HSE do not expect the design team to become obsessed with the subject. Design team members need to be free to explore and develop their thinking unfettered. Focusing on the potential risks of materials or construction techniques at too early a stage can devalue the design.

Instead, the team members should focus on fulfilling the Project Objectives and then, if necessary, developing safe and practical solutions to constructing the design.

### Examples of design development

#### The potential problem: large components

A design includes large timber windows as a feature, but they are heavy and cannot be safely manually installed. Planning consent favours the window design and significant change would cause delays. Can the team produce a design and installation approach that will minimise and control the potential risks?

The problem needs to be broken down into the key issues:

– Can the windows be broken down into several sub-units? The first design option is to look at smaller units. This is possible, but it will introduce many more joint tolerances to be controlled, installation may take longer and the potential for failure of weather sealing is increased.
– Can they be mechanically installed, keeping the design as a set of large windows and arranging for a wholly mechanical installation? Equipment designed to place components in difficult locations is available, but will need to be researched by the design team. Simple sketches of the proposed erection sequence can help at this stage, as can advice from specialist installers or contractors.

Mechanical installation does have limits and once tested it has to be ruled out as the site is too constricted for mechanical handling. The window design therefore progresses with smaller units, which are to be assembled on site. As this will affect the detailed design tendering and the choice of manufacturer this analysis needs to

## Examples of design development (*continued*)

be done ahead of procurement. This process has to be noted in the project files, but requires no more than an explanation of the issues, the potential risks and how they have been addressed.

The smaller units match the original design and are easily within the safe capabilities of two men to install. The need for careful weathertight assembly must be communicated to the on-site team. The team agree this is the right answer for everyone.

The construction sequence and larger number of windows mean that installation will take slightly longer. The contractor needs to take account of this in the construction programme. This may also increase the cost, so the client needs to be made aware of the process the design team have undertaken, justifying the increase in cost and time.

### The potential problem: excessive cutting on site

A courtyard between existing buildings is to be paved and planters constructed in the middle. The client wants heavy Portland stone to be used. The design calls for a symmetrical layout starting from the planters and includes crossfalls and drainage channels. As a result, a large percentage of the slabs need to be cut on site.

What options exist to minimise and control the harmful effects of on-site cutting?

– Step back from the design and look at simplification. Perhaps create two lines of symmetry, one either side of the planters: large areas can be the same, and with careful on-site measurement most slabs can be cut off site.
– Avoid any crossfalls and incorporate drainage channels into the pattern of joints.
– Given the set boundaries created by the existing buildings, the junctions between the paving and the buildings need to be flexible. Perhaps introduce a new design element, such as gravel or planting, to eliminate the need to cut slabs at boundaries.
– Ensure mechanical placement equipment can be used.

All of these measures should be noted in the project records, and the client must be kept informed of the decisions and the reasons behind them.

## Opportunities and risks

At this stage, while there is fluidity in the design, there are opportunities to improve the health and safety of the scheme. However, new issues can emerge that have the potential to cause problems later on.

The principal elements of the project need to be considered at this stage, such as ensuring that the geometry and site layout allow for complete facade access by one means or another. These will not be fully detailed at this stage, but the space or conceptual approach needs to be included within the Concept Design. If such elements are not addressed at this stage, major health and safety issues can be 'locked into' the Concept Design, creating the need to revisit Stage 2 during Stages 3 or 4.

A plan is needed to ensure that, as the design is progressively fixed, it is checked for health and safety implications. Using the structure of the project to ensure these aspects are covered where necessary and recorded is key. Administration should be kept simple – just enough to help stay on track. It is important that any issues are recorded immediately as they develop – attempting to recount what has happened, even a few days later, often results in inaccurate recording.

Sometimes the best designs take the team into completely new territory. This is obviously challenging, but it can be very rewarding. Making clear what the issues are and encouraging the team to come up with answers can be stressful, but often results in the very best solutions.

### Modular construction

It is worth considering modular construction, where the majority of construction is carried out off site. Modules of complete rooms – especially where there is a high degree of repetition, such as in hotels – are prime targets for this methodology. While this will mean craning large and heavy components onto site, this process can be closely controlled and, when undertaken by skilled operators, has minimal risks.

### Assemblies

Increasingly, preassembled building elements are seen as having many advantages for health and safety. While modular construction involves the process of bringing near completed parts together on site, this technique involves smaller components.

## Modular plant

Several significant City of London office developments have used preassembled modular plant units. These are assembled, tested and quality checked in the factory before being transported to site. While there is increased risk when installing the relatively large and heavy modules on site, significant risks are removed due to the reduced number of site operations and need for work in confined space or work involving a large number of electrical or high-pressure components.

While improving health and safety, this has also improved reliability, quality and installation time.

For complex or otherwise onerous parts of the design, this can be a significantly safer approach, and one that also delivers better quality and requires less time on site.

## Airport arrivals piers

Roofing elements and air circulation ductwork assemblies complete with grilles and connections have been used at Gatwick airport to shorten construction time and reduce the amount of high-level working on piers.

### Process focused v design focused

As the Concept Design starts to develop there is a tendency to ignore the 'how' and to focus entirely on the 'what'. While this is understandable – the 'what' will be reflected in the finished building, but the 'how' will be short lived and may only be of importance during construction – it should be resisted.

Often the 'what' (a physical element of the construction, such as a window) is readily identified and easily understood from the health and safety aspect. It is more difficult to understand the health and safety implications of the 'how' (manufacturing, procurement, transportation to site and assembly). Often the full implications of assembling the many components in the right order and ensuring they all come together as intended is complex and requires the full range of experience across the complete team. Sharing the different perspectives of the team is often a good way to ensure this is completely understood. How well this is undertaken directly affects the buildability when the project goes to site. Coordination of the design and information to form one coherent message with equal emphasis on the what and how is a mark of high-quality health and safety methodology.

It is vital that designers consider process. The range of processes will be determined by how components are assembled on site. Are they necessarily the ones that fit with the project strategy? Are there any better options with fewer hazards, such as sourcing of natural materials with better characteristics? What processes have to be undertaken on site? Can they be improved to be less hazardous by using a different design, a different approach or even different materials?

### Focus on process

Paviours and kerbs are designed to be assembled on site, which inevitably involves some cutting. However, cutting of these materials is dangerous and can be very unhealthy for the operatives unless all the controls are followed. It would be so much better if the design and the following construction processes could ensure that no cutting on site is needed.

## Finalising the Concept Design

At the end of Stage 2, the design principles should be clear and many of the key features – covering the structure, the massing, the general layout and the materials – will have been determined.

The key decisions are likely to have come about after many iterations of the design. At each iteration there should have been a systematic review and filtering of health and safety issues. The design team should have considered how the design will be procured and constructed, including options such as off-site manufacturing, and given a clear description of any harmful aspects. Any risks that have not been designed out should have been identified, so they can be kept under consideration at the next stage.

At this point there will be many issues that have yet to be fully developed. There will be many areas where generic products have been identified but are yet to be narrowed down. The assessments therefore need to be kept open, with a degree of tolerance over what to rule in and what to rule out based on difficultly or risk.

If a planning application is to be made at the end of Stage 2, the Concept Design should be sufficiently developed to allow its submission. Some design elements required for the planning application need to be fully thought through, including any health and safety implications. Often this is truly the start of procurement and can benefit from the input from a contractor or specialists from the supply chain.

Cost Information begins to be defined during this stage and must take account of potential health and safety issues.

The Final Project Brief will also be prepared at the end of this stage, capturing any changes from the Initial Project Brief that have resulted from the preparation of the Concept Design.

## Stage 2 checklist

- Has the client been informed of their responsibilities under the CDM regulations?
- Has the client confirmed they are aware of their responsibilities?
- Has the form F10 (where applicable) been submitted to the HSE?
- Has the team been made aware of the Health and Safety Strategy?
- Is the design being developed in a proportionate and balanced manner?
- Does the team have a process for recording key decisions?
- Does the team have a process for recording risks not yet resolved?
- Is there an emerging understanding of the construction processes?
- Has the health and safety file been set up?
- Has the client been kept up to date by regular reporting at team meetings?

## Information Exchanges

Information Exchanges required for Stage 2 are as follows:

| at stage completion: the Concept Design, including outline structural and building services design and associated Project Strategies, preliminary Cost Information and Final Project Brief
| for UK Government projects: an output of Project Information is required.

## Chapter summary 2

During Stage 2 the requirements of the Initial Project Brief will be developed into a fully rounded Concept Design, and a revised Final Project Brief will be prepared. It is vital that the Health and Safety Strategy continues to be developed, setting the standards for stages to come.

Procedures and systems should be fully set up and fed into the project as required. The design process must get off to a proper start at this stage, therefore it is important that no shortcuts are taken. Corrective procedures should be in place in case shortcuts do start to creep in.

Many options and variations may be present during this stage; ensuring that all the implications of each are understood can be challenging. It may also be difficult to make the case for health and safety concerns. In many ways the Concept Design stage is the most challenging for the design team: as the design emerges, the designers must ensure there is a balance between risk and design, and an understanding of the processes that will be needed. Experience, understanding and preparation are vital.

Projecting the full picture of the emerging design and related construction sequence is necessary and making sure this is part of the project decision-making process is critical.

It is essential to take note of the (town) planning, programme and procurement strategies and to ensure that the whole team are aware of all health and safety aspects emerging from these.

Key points to remember during Stage 2:

| Every iteration of the Concept Design will have health and safety implications.
| Make sure during the design development that there is awareness across the team.
| At the Concept Design stage it is easy to forget construction implications.
| Ensure that all design reviews address health and safety.
| Simple, clear processes keep everyone 'on board'.
| Make sure the design outcomes properly address any practical issues.
| At this stage there is no need to focus on detail: it's big picture items that are important.

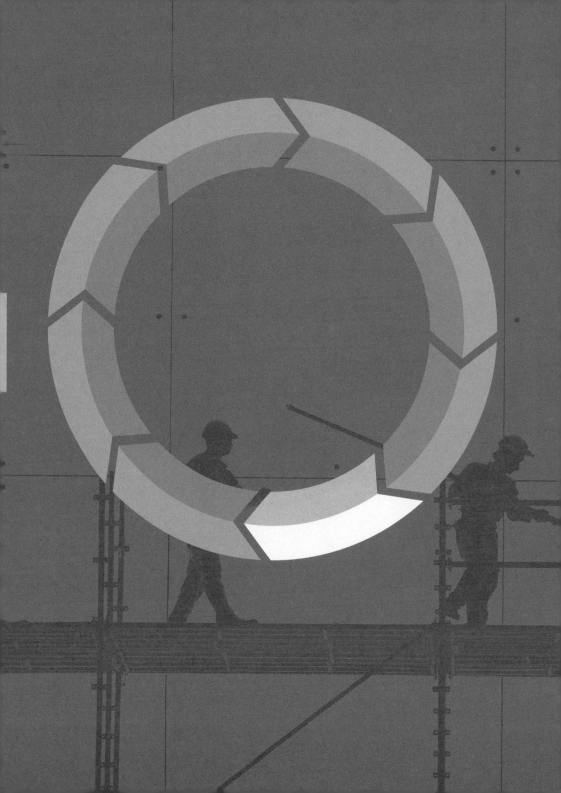

# Developed Design

# Chapter overview

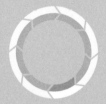

Stage 3 is a critical point in a project in terms of health and safety considerations, as detail emerges and earlier assumptions are clarified. Decisions made now are increasingly difficult to change. As the design is developed and coordinated, careful consideration of how the detail will develop during Stage 4 is required. The Construction Strategy should be reviewed and updated, with the emerging refined health and safety requirements being an intrinsic element.

For this stage, the Core Objectives focus around the lead designer coordinating the work of the design team. Developed proposals for the structural design, building services systems and outline specifications are prepared. Cost Information is updated and the Project Strategies fleshed out. The design team may be expanded, perhaps with the addition of a health and safety adviser.

With respect to town planning applications, this is the most likely stage for the application to be made. Once the application is submitted, some of the project characteristics will, to all intents and purposes, become fixed.

Where they apply, the CDM regulations will continue to influence the management of risk on the project.

**The key coverage in this chapter is as follows:**

Core activities at this stage

Key health and safety tasks at Stage 3

The health and safety file

The project team and health and safety

Exchange of health and safety information
_____

Product processes and issues
_____

Further considerations at this stage
_____

BIM (and health and safety)
_____

Operation and maintenance
_____

Information Exchanges
_____

# Introduction

It is important to recognise that, at Stage 3, aspects of the design start to become fixed and so issues that have impacts on health and safety must be considered carefully. The Developed Design, including structural, mechanical and electrical design, requires a significant level of detail to be added to the Project Information. In developing that detail, the team must consider the health and safety implications in parallel with everything else as the design is progressed, continuing to use the method of working established in previous stages.

The team must adopt an approach that ensures significant decisions are recorded, clearly spelling out their design approach. In particular, any unusual issues must be highlighted, especially if they appear to be unique to the project.

Specification details will be developed during this stage. Ideally, these will have begun to be defined early in Stage 2. During Stage 3, the majority of the detail will be added, defined or identified, much of which may relate to products identified for inclusion within the project. As with other areas of technical design, in developing the specification, health and safety issues must always be considered as an integrated part of the design process. The specification can include guidance on risk mitigation, working procedures and process requirements, which can all help to ensure good practice.

Cost Information should be developed in parallel with the specification. Significant tensions often develop between the specification and the defined level of performance and cost. The team need to carefully review these aspects and ensure the balance is right, using the most accurate information that can be accessed. This cost versus performance evaluation often needs to be revisited during Stage 4, so making robust decisions at this stage can help to avoid very difficult issues later.

The debate between specification and cost often has significant health and safety implications. These should be flagged up for the attention of the client and sensibly debated within the team. Solutions can often be found that ensure there are no negative outcomes, but these require careful consideration and the involvement of the full team to be achieved effectively.

Project strategies that have been carefully formulated in previous stages need to be checked regularly to ensure they reflect the current design direction.

### From Stage 2

It is also important to take full advantage of the Stage 2 preparations.

Ensure the client understands the principles being developed.

Ensure the team is developing the design in line with the Project Objectives.

Ensure the Concept Design principles are robust and still minimise risk.

## What are the Core Objectives of this stage?

The Core Objectives of the RIBA Plan of Work 2013 at Stage 3 are:

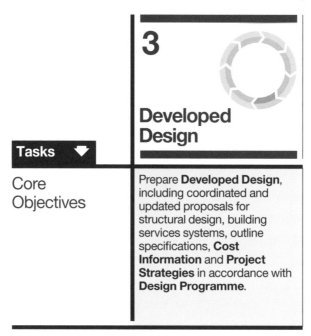

The Core Objectives at this stage involve all design team members developing the design so that it is coordinated. The layout, structural design, building services design, the Sustainability Strategy, the cost and key Project Strategies all take a significant step towards the Technical Design used to construct and then maintain the building. Several significant areas are addressed during this stage, principally planning, technical strategies (Building Regulations approaches), cost and defined performance, making this a critical and complex stage.

## Core activities at this stage

The core activities at this stage are to ensure that the early assumptions are validated and achievable (or are removed) and are fed into the project design. This stage of design development requires further levels of information, to support the principles of the project established in earlier stages. This will almost certainly include product information, process information and specific finishes and fittings for the first time.

As any Research and Development activities are concluded and the design is refined, it is essential that any new information is reviewed from a health and safety perspective and added to the Project Information. This can be a very straightforward process – it does not need to be overly intensive or a diversion away from other tasks. Having a clear methodology is helpful in this respect. This methodology should include a focus on the level of detail – an increasingly important concept, especially where BIM is used – which should be consistent across all disciplines.

Each design team member will have information relating to design in the form of original drawn or written requirements. Products, performance requirements, standards and possibly entire specification sections will be under development at this time. These will all be based on earlier outline information, but will increasingly be taking shape and moving closer to becoming the completed Project Information.

### Design review example

The design calls for large module slate flooring to be used in the entrance hall. Each slate would be very heavy and difficult to move into place. The design needs to be reviewed to determine whether the size of unit is critical or if it can be reduced to a more manageable size. Looking at the overall design, other elements, such as the curtain walling, match the slate size. Bearing in mind the difficulties for installation, it is agreed to go ahead with the size as originally designed.

The design team then work with a specialist supplier to develop a safe and practical method of delivery and installation. At Stage 4, a drawing installation plan will be produced and elements added to the specification and a recommended method of work added to the pre-construction documents.

The principal designer must ensure that all team members work together and produce sensible solutions. As previously mentioned, overuse of the terms 'coordinate' and 'cooperate' (from the EU directive) has considerably devalued their effect. Perhaps a better term to use for design information is that it must be 'coherent and robust'.

## Planning application

At this stage a town planning application will often be made. It is important to recognise that details included within the application may have health and safety implications. Once consent has been given, the geometry, layout and materials, and perhaps even access, maintenance and cleaning options, will be fixed.

Prior to an application being submitted, these areas need to be reviewed. They should be discussed with the client and safe options found for construction and use of the project. Consideration of site layout, general massing, materials and cleaning and maintenance will be included in the planning application deliverables. In granting consent, planning authorities often deem these points to be conditioned; as such, the health and safety implications must be understood in advance of the application being made. After planning consent is granted there will be only limited room for change.

It is often considered a significant milestone when planning consent is granted. As many options are fixed from this point, the design team need to be clear that the options they are left with are ones where risk has been assessed, understood and minimised.

## Risk identification and reduction

As design is progressed and decisions are being made, each team member needs to look carefully at their design in terms of potential risk. The issues created by unusual or complex designs and assemblies must be considered to reduce or remove any risks.

All design team members must share their designs to ensure coordination between the design disciplines. At this stage, issues can arise that had not been apparent previously; for instance, when the architectural detail is amalgamated with the structural design. As each of the team members develops their design, which in turn is assimilated into one set of information, further review is necessary to allow new risks to be identified. This process may have to be undertaken several times to ensure all potential risks that may be generated between disciplines are identified.

If possible, all health and safety risks should be designed out. If they cannot be removed, then they should be minimised and flagged up for special attention, with clear information provided to prevent any surprises during construction. Where there are remaining risks, the design team must be able to offer at least one safe and practical method of construction. Liaison with construction specialists at this point may be necessary. In fact, even when the design team are confident that no such problems remain in the design, it is well worth having the design reviewed from a contractor's perspective. This could be by the potential principal contractor, or by one employed specifically for this limited activity.

These considerations apply equally to all design phases of the project. From this stage on – through the procurement, construction, handover, in use and, finally, demolition phases – it is essential to keep the details under continuous review for emerging hazards.

### Safe rooftop access

The Concept Design might include a requirement for safe rooftop access, to allow maintenance and repair of the building fabric and the rooftop plant. The design team will then have to consider the risks involved and how they can be minimised. One solution would be to use rooftop railings, but these will often be a challenge for designers and are disliked by planners. Another option would be to continue the fabric of the building above roof level to form an 'invisible parapet'. This increases the cost of the fabric, but allows safe access to the whole roof area. Many clients see the advantage of this approach, not only in terms of safety but also in the provision of a roof terrace – good health and safety delivering value for money as well.

Alternatively, designing a full screen around all of the regularly accessed areas of the roof can also be successful. A full-height louvered wall can be employed, making the plant access safe for maintenance staff. Access outside this area, which will only be needed for roof and cladding repairs, should be limited to operatives with full protective equipment and training.

## Procurement

As the level of detail in the Developed Design increases, exactly how the various components will be procured becomes clearer. As this becomes established, the potential for increased or changed risks that could affect other elements needs to be checked.

Products and components of a conventional nature can be sourced to suit the contractor's supply chain and will be predictable. Specialised product systems and components, however, may have to come from a limited or unique source and must be analysed for any risk creation issues.

The design team need to be alive to any changes in the sourcing of components or materials that could throw up increased or changed risks. For example, changing a steel lintel to a concrete one might not affect performance but could have implications for handling.

## Team structure

For the team to work efficiently and in a managed way, its structure needs to be clear and understood by all members. The Design Responsibilities Matrix and the Contractual Tree will define this structure, but a project organogram should also have been drafted at Stage 1 and updated at Stage 2. These now need a further review.

## Updating the Health and Safety Strategy

The Health and Safety Strategy recommended under the RIBA Plan of Work 2013 elevates the subject to a more prominent position. Without a formal strategy, it can be easy to overlook health and safety during the early project stages.

The Health and Safety Strategy – along with the other key Project Strategies – must be reviewed and updated during each project stage. At Stage 3, the majority of considerations will be in relation to the CDM regulations. However, it is important to take as wide a view of health and safety as possible – not just focusing on regulatory compliance.

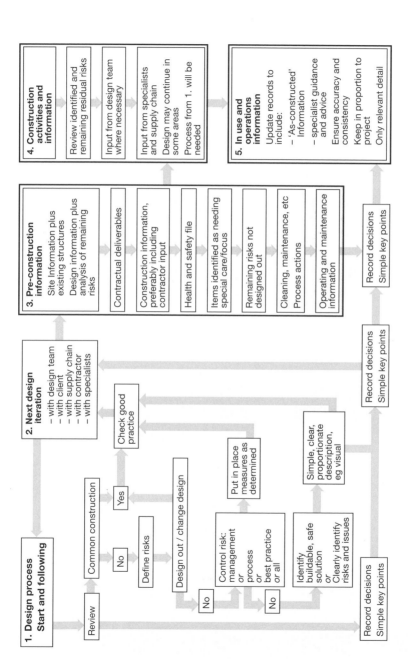

*Figure 3.1  CDM risk analysis*

## Key health and safety tasks at Stage 3

The following tasks are key to the successful completion of Stage 3:

| Confirm the client understands their duties

The first person to be appointed as designer has the responsibility to ensure the client understands their duties (see page 55: Stage 1). However, it is always worthwhile checking that the client has been made aware of their duties by the lead consultant, the principal designer or, on a very small project, the principal contractor.

| Confirm the client is aware of progress

Some clients are fully engaged with the project, some are only focused on delivery and cost, but all need to be made aware of health and safety. Beyond Stage 3, it becomes increasingly difficult to make changes to the design and so health and safety issues that are allowed to go beyond this point unchallenged may be difficult to correct later. The team leader needs to ensure that regular reporting on health and safety to the client is in place.

| Confirm all required processes are in place

After the design development, a check across all project processes is recommended. Pressures within the project can often lead to these being watered down or bypassed. This is a good point at which to reaffirm what is expected – the team leader should cover this at a project team meeting.

| Confirm the project has been notified to the HSE

If notification is required under the CDM regulations, confirm that a form F10 has been issued. While this is the client's responsibility, it will often fall to the team leader, principal designer or health and safety specialist to make the F10 submission.

| Ensure all team members are signed up to a consistent set of procedures

It cannot be emphasised enough that ensuring the team members are working together is essential. By the time Stage 3 comes around, working habits will be established. The lead designer should ensure that procedures are in place and that they reflect what was agreed at the start of the project.

| Ensure the principal designer role is in place and working
It is the client's responsibility to ensure the principal designer role is established. It is essential that this is checked at this stage.

| Ensure that all health and safety considerations are relevant and proportionate to the project
At the detailed development stage, health and safety considerations can multiply out of control. This is as bad as paying too little attention to this area as the most significant issues can be buried within the paperwork. A proportionate approach is therefore essential. The team leader should drive this, with support from the client.

## Practice Note: Check your procedures

Sometimes, when projects have been running for a while, there can be a tendency for enhancements to methods of working and procedures to creep in and for additional requirements to be added, often without any real thought as to how effective they are. Adding an additional layer of risk analysis or an extra check on materials is only effective if it brings a provable benefit. To test whether the procedures being used are appropriate, take one simple example and work it through. Can the current methodology be improved? If not, leave it alone – the simplest procedure is nearly always the best.

For example, the current procedures might give the following analysis:

– Does the design require the use of cut bricks?
– Can cut bricks be removed from the design?
– What would be the implications for the design: costs, aesthetics, buildability?
– Can the number of cut bricks be reduced?
– Can pre-cut bricks be sourced?
– Can on-site cutting of bricks be avoided?

Can the procedures be changed to improve on this analysis? For example:

– Design everything to conform to standard brick dimensions. However, this might reduce flexibility, change the aesthetics and require changes to other components.
– Discuss alternatives with a brick specialist or the contractor.

## Practice Note: Check your procedures (*continued*)

These are practical enhancements, but equally the following changes could be considered:

– Review every brick detail.
– Change the risk analysis procedure.
– Add a requirement to the specification that brick cutting is to be avoided.
– Develop detailed procedures for safe cutting on site.

In this case, it is likely that none of these changes would result in an improvement over the procedures already in place.

## Things to watch out for at this stage

### Too much paperwork

Every member of the team needs to reflect on the amount of information they produce (in any media). All information needs to be focused and relevant if it is to be effective.

### Reinterpretation

All too often, requirements can become redefined – especially those concerning health and safety – usually resulting in them seeming more complex or onerous. In response, the HSE set up its Myth Busters Challenge Panel to help dispel common misconceptions.

A recent example is the reinterpretation of the requirements for electrical testing of portable appliances. Many people have become convinced that annual testing is a legal requirement – as a result, an industry has grown up around annual testing of all appliances. However, this is not required under any regulations. Appliances only need to be properly maintained, and tested for electrical safety when changes are made or a fault is suspected.

It is difficult to establish where these reinterpretations start, but the cautious team will always refer back to the HSE if they have any doubts.

## Things to watch out for at this stage (*continued*)

### A client wants their procedures used

Working with a receptive client can be a joy; some clients, however, expect the team to work to their methodologies and procedures. While it is reasonable to expect repeat clients to have their own ways of working, some have developed bad habits or systems that do not necessarily fit well with health and safety legislation. All team members need to be aware of this potential.

The lead designer should conduct a walk-through of the client's procedures and consider how they affect the team's roles and remit. This may result in a gentle conversation with the client being required. Most clients will be open to suggestions and welcome improvements, but some may need a firmer hand. Putting concerns in writing is always recommended – explaining the seriousness of the issue can, most of the time, bring the client around. Ultimately, keep your professional indemnity insurer informed, and if there is a serious problem it may be sensible to resign the commission.

### Simple wins

All members of the team need to be on the lookout for simple wins. In a commercial world, where value for money, efficient working and ensuring you're on top make all the difference, any sort of simple innovation can prove immensely valuable.

For example, most health and safety issues are far better expressed in a drawing or other visual format – quick to understand, quick to communicate and normally quick to resolve.

### Good intentions

Good intentions can be both a positive and a negative. All too often, good intentions – attempting to work for the greater good – can come unhinged if not properly structured and backed by the right experience. It is better to adopt a cautious approach. As is so often said, if it looks too good to be true, it probably is. It is always better to stand back a little and take a wider, more considered view, than to rush into something that appears obvious. Health and safety is not something you want to get wrong.

### Least cost v value for money

The challenge of balancing least cost and value for money is one that runs right across any project. So often, least cost turns out to

**Things to watch out for at this stage (*continued*)**

be poor value for money, but it may take time for this to become obvious, at which point it is too late to correct.

Especially in the health and safety elements of the project, it is critical that chasing least cost does not affect decision-making. At this stage, when design actions are becoming fixed, it is essential that the project leaders can apply a firm hand. For example, value engineering exercises often lead to safety equipment being removed from the design. The reason usually given is that the equipment is to be provided from a separate maintenance budget. In nearly every case it is never installed, leaving maintenance staff exposed to unnecessary and illegal risks.

## The health and safety file

Under the CDM regulations, the production of the health and safety file is a key responsibility of the principal designer (see page 149: Stage 4). The file's purpose is to provide all the key information that others – the contractor, the building owner and the building users – may need to ensure a safe understanding of the design. If for any reason this is not done, the responsibility falls to the client.

The file should have been started during Stage 2 and developed since that point. However, it is often not until this stage that substantial content is added due to the outline and iterative nature of the Project Information. The principal designer will require the assistance of the whole design team to keep the file updated.

Remember the following key points when updating the file:

I Keeping it up to date saves time later and makes it more accurate.
I Only relevant information in proportion to the project should be included.
I Avoid lengthy text. There should only be explanations.
I Contemporaneous notes are always helpful, to aid memory later.

One of the best ways to keep everything up to date is to have prepared some simple but relevant templates. These can be used on every project and are easy to keep updated. They can be issued as interim reports and can be invaluable for quick reference.

### Templates

Use templates for all repetitive CDM activities. They can be as simple as a table formatted to the office standard. Templates for the following are suggested as a minimum:

- design issues identified
- residual risks to be passed on
- details of a particular issue, including drawn details, to be passed on.

## The project team and health and safety

It is important that all project team members understand the need for the Health and Safety Strategy to work across the project team as a whole. In order to achieve this, the essential ingredients of good management apply. For clarity these are included below.

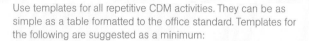

### Dealing with design changes

Change Control Procedures begin in earnest at Stage 3. Change as a result of design development and external influences is inevitable, but it needs to be accounted for and controlled, especially within the design team. How this happens will develop considerably in the future, as BIM-driven projects become more widespread.

Control of change is needed so that established principles are not watered down, safe methodologies do not become risk laden and errors do not creep in, generating what can become serious on-site hazards. As design detail becomes richer, there is more to consider: in many respects, the level of complexity is increasing rapidly. However, the picture can remain clear, as long as the team have a focused appreciation of what is current.

Changes can often be the cause of unconsidered or uncoordinated information. Thinking through the unintended consequences of any change is just as important as thinking through the intended consequences. For example, using a different size of component because it is easier to transport, handle and get to site may also mean it needs to be cut or fixed together on site, creating a new set of hazards.

Equally, it might take some time before the knock-on effects of a change emerge. Considering the full implications of any change is challenging but necessary. This is where experience counts. From this point on in the project, change is always pressured and nearly always time constrained giving even more reason to enforce rigid Change Control Procedures.

**Principles for Change Control Procedures**

Change control involves the adoption of some basic processes used in the quality assurance world.

The Project Information first needs to be baselined; that is to say, a consolidated, checked, verified and organised set of information is established for the project. This should be regarded as the reference documentation. Many clients like this approach because it gives a sense of control that might otherwise be lacking.

From the point that the baselined information is established and issued, a change management system is introduced across the project. Under the RIBA Plan of Work 2013, this involves the adoption of a set of Change Control Procedures, which will apply to all changes, irrespective of who has instigated them or why. It is normal for either the client, the project manager or the architect to issue a process map for the procedures. This will need to be adhered to throughout the remaining stages of the project.

If for any reason a change to the baselined information is thought to be needed, the project team member responsible will have to prepare a change control document. This will identify the change and all the pertinent facts surrounding it, including who is calling for the change, any possible cost and time implications and, of course, any health and safety issues. This document will be circulated for comment and possible approval across the whole project team. The change cannot progress until all the team agree and the document has been signed off by the client.

Where the prospective change affects work within a tender package, this can cause difficulties. Otherwise, it is an effective way of managing changes that, if not controlled, could easily result in risks accumulating in specific areas of the project.

## Change control

The principles of change management are explained in
BS EN ISO 9004:2009 *Managing for the sustained success of an
organization.*

### Coordinating the design team information

Key information needs to be coordinated across the design team on a
regular basis, so that it will be robust and coherent. It is essential that all
members of the team are aware of each other's information in order to
understand how it will come together. In a BIM environment, this is made
obvious to all members of the team. The use of BIM can help to prevent
clashes arising in the design and ensure there is design continuity. It
will also improve health and safety, as sequences can be analysed and
risks reviewed. Clashes discovered late in the day are always a source
of added risk.

### Information quality and delivery

It is essential that information is issued in a timely manner and that it is
clear and unambiguous. Lack of clarity can have an impact on health
and safety. There is an absolute need for clarity to avoid misconceptions,
to head off problems on site and to ensure the team members are fully
coordinated in their thinking.

The design information needs to show the contractor exactly what is
intended. If a detailed point of the design cannot be explained for any
reason, the information should say so, thus allowing the contractor to make
a reasonable assessment of what is needed. Poor quality information
leaves it up to the site staff to interpret what is required, which can result
in unsafe or risk-laden work – it will not be possible to make adequate
site preparations or ensure that the correct equipment and skills are
available.

## Getting the most out of the design team

### Why are simple, clear procedures important?

The average small project will require at least five design team members to be involved for most of the time. There is every likelihood this number will be supplemented intermittently, as others become involved. The contractor will consist of an equal number of subcontractors, and this is in addition to the client and their team. As a result, considerable effort will be required to ensure the information as developed is consistent across this team.

### What does this entail?

Attention to detail and consistent management is needed. There must be good inter-team relationships and everyone must have a clearly defined responsibility to ensure they are up to date and are keeping everyone else in the project team up to date about project and industry issues.

### Keep control

Whatever position they hold in the project team, there is a need for all project team members to stay ahead of the information flow and keep control of what is current. If they are in a position of authority, such as the project lead or lead designer, this is much more important. The project and the client rely on senior management to ensure success.

### Ensure all issues are covered

Ensuring there is comprehensive coverage of all the information on a project can be challenging. Even on smaller projects, it can be difficult just to maintain an awareness of its range and scope. Good procedures and robust controls keep this manageable. All information must be registered and all issued deliverables must be version controlled.

### Use simple, pre-agreed procedures

The methodology, templates and procedures set up for the practice now come fully into their own. Make them work for you when you come to this technical stage. Often, when well-managed companies come together in a team – each with its own procedures – they will agree early on which company's procedures will take precedence on the project. Mixing procedures or not having a clear agreement is not advised.

**Getting the most out of the team (*continued*)**

**To safeguard future decisions, record the past**
While the essence of good health and safety is avoiding excessive paperwork, you need to safeguard future decisions. Ensure there are contemporaneous notes of key decisions. This is especially important on projects that run over several years.

## Exchange of health and safety information

### Concise content

It is nearly always the case, despite good planning, that resources are stretched on any project. It is therefore important that, as the volume of information increases, it is well managed. It also needs to be efficiently delivered. If not, errors can easily creep in that will rapidly erode all the good work achieved.

It should only be necessary to produce a relatively small amount of information related solely to health and safety. A substantial proportion of Project Information, if well structured and presented, will contain implicit health and safety information. Some dedicated health and safety information is needed from a regulatory perspective. This will revolve around the health and safety file, the development of essential maintenance information and ensuring the background decision-making has been captured.

### Principles for good information exchange

The overriding principle is to keep information clear and explicit. For purposes of health and safety it is much better to use drawn or visual references wherever possible. At Stage 3, when a lot of the project detail is clear, the information can be expressed as a cross-project matrix (see appendix 3), with additional, more detailed reference sheets linked to it.

Doubling-up on the use of drawings – so they serve more than one purpose – is ideal here. CAD applications use the principle of multi-layer drawings – in a similar way, hazard analysis or hazard communication can be considered as just another layer. Even when working with single-layer CAD, this can be a useful way of thinking about any health and safety information. This helps the designer to focus on identifying the important issues.

## Hard copy

Hard copy has been the traditional way of providing information, and for some it is still the preferred and usual practice. Ensure that your hard copy has followed the normal good practice principles – that every document is referenced and every issue is recorded on the document and elsewhere in the project records. In these records, make clear what the document is and why it has been issued.

Always keep a correctly filed exact copy of issued documents in the office, in a separate health and safety project file (not to be confused with the health and safety file required for CDM purposes).

## Electronic information

The vast majority of information is communicated in an electronic format. The controls used for hard copy documents apply equally to electronic information.

Along with the advantages of speed and easy duplication come the issues of correct transmission and editing. Every document issued should be sent in an uneditable format, but accompanied by a duplicate document in an editable format. Any editable information is issued for use by the recipient at their own risk.

## Identify areas of consideration

At this stage the design should be well advanced with significant detail included. Except on the smallest of projects, this will have been produced by a number of authors, perhaps from different companies. It is often the responsibility of the lead designer, or perhaps the architect, the project manager or maybe the client's representative, to review and comment on the information as a whole.

| It is important for the efficiency of the Construction Programme that every detail agrees with every other.

❘ There may be a range of different options to consider, so it is important to ensure that they have all been considered. It can be easy to overlook alternative options in the pressure to issue information.

## Product processes and issues

Specific products will often be specified during this stage. However, the choice of particular products can raise a number of issues for the design team.

❘ Compatibility
The biggest potential issue is the interrelationship between bespoke products and purpose-designed elements, so checks will have to be made to ensure they are compatible and to demonstrate good buildability.

❘ Product hazards
Issues here can relate to size, weight or a specific hazard, such as sharp edges, electrical hazards or even chemical risk. For example, a great deal can be done by the team around dimensions alone. Check that dimensions given are for the 'as delivered' product. Can items of this size be handled by normal procedures, or will special equipment be needed to move them to the work site?

❘ Repetitive operations
A product that comprises a large number of small components can be equally challenging and provision should be made for a safe method of installation. Requiring site operatives to carry out repetitive operations over long periods can cause significant injury. The design team may therefore have to devise a novel working method.

❘ Handling of materials
The movement and cutting of materials are two of the most challenging and potentially hazardous issues confronted by site personnel. Hazards such as this are often invisible to the design team as design team members are rarely present on site. Large quantities of cutting or reworking can have serious implications on site, especially if significant equipment or temporary works are required.

The team must make it their job to identify detailed information concerning assembly and fixing details before deciding on a particular product.

Unfortunately, components are often chosen without realising they will be impossible to install safely, which unnecessarily increases the pressure on the construction team. The details of specified products should be added to the Project Information, including their intended performance and construction sequence.

### Review and record products

- Not all product information is consistent and clear – make comparisons with care.
- Develop a method for reviewing products and take forward the findings so that detail is not lost.
- Record each product's essential details and copy them into the health and safety file.
- A spreadsheet of all products being considered may be the most practical method for capturing the details.
- Electronic forms of specification can also be helpful.

### Buildability

Buildability and the issues that it generates are often the subject of some debate within project teams. Potential buildability issues (buildability is largely about health and safety) are the core of the practical considerations needed in design. It is essential to check buildability issues on a regular basis at design and client meetings (see also page 151: Stage 4).

### Temporary works

Temporary works are commonly required for structural elements, but they can also be needed for mechanical and electrical services, fire prevention or traffic routing, or even for ensuring that a client's business operations are maintained during the construction processes. At this stage, requirements for any temporary works should be emerging, if not already formulated.

With the design developed, these can now be thought through to the same level as the main project. They should be planned within the main project and have the same degree of analysis and organisation as any other part of the project. The structural engineer will often lead in this area, but it is crucial that all members of the design team understand the implications for their work and that they contribute to the dialogue. The team have a responsibility under the CDM regulations to ensure the contractor is offered a well-considered temporary works design that is as risk free as possible.

## Further considerations at this stage

Except on the most straightforward projects, there will always be some issues that can be considered special or unusual. The challenge for project teams generally is that every project is unique and has it own special challenges.

Any special issues should have emerged during this stage, so any health and safety concerns can be clearly identified and considered. Any documents being used to track these issues need to be up to date and reflect the latest understanding.

Most of the time it will be sufficient to devote a little team resource to examining these issues in finer detail and coming up with a plan for dealing with them, which is then fed back into the Project Information. In this way, others will be well aware of the issues and able to take appropriate action, especially during construction.

### Exceptional issues

Issues that need special consideration could include:

- the need to divert a river during construction
- the need to move a client's business centre so that their business can continue to function
- the presence of complex or highly sensitive infrastructure nearby.

### Site arrangements

In Stages 1 and 2 some thought, from a health and safety perspective, will have been given to the arrangements for site operations. It is important that these are reviewed during this stage. The aim is not to take over from the construction team, but for the design team to contribute positively to a safer project.

## BIM (and health and safety)

In Stage 3, when Project Information has become much more reliable and detailed, the Building Information Modelling (BIM) approach will really start to deliver significant benefits. BIM methodologies help ensure the developed design can be reviewed across the project team, and that its implications are spelt out to the client, the contractor and, possibly, regulators.

At the time of writing, a range of BIM techniques, software and approaches are being developed – especially for the health and safety areas. From demonstration projects undertaken to date it is clear that BIM will make considerable advances possible, taking health and safety to a different level of processing and allowing decisions to be made with confidence across the team. However, this does depend on the development of adequate and joined-up data.

BIM data is well developed by Stage 3 and robust and reliable data will be available for analysis. As design details are added, graphical analysis can be used to show three-dimensional relationships. A BIM model is capable of assembling components in the sequence of construction. The design team can use this to identify any hazards created by the construction process. Currently, it is only possible to assess the design and the components for possible hazards; in time, improved software will allow real time review as well. Buildability can also be checked using the BIM model.

Specialist software is currently being developed to flag up critical relationships in the design, so that the design team can consider suitable alternatives. This real-time checking will not be limited to health and safety; issues relating to compliance with other regulations can be dealt with at the same time.

The BIM model data can also be reviewed for risk issues by using filters. For instance, it can be searched for abnormal shapes, weights or chemical content. Any potential hazards will be flagged up for the design team.

Hopefully, the BIM model will confirm that there will be no problems if the design and construction sequence are followed, in which case it can be used as a record that this is the case.

Within this verification process compliance with the regulations and, in turn, the health and safety profile will be reviewed and clearly reported to the client. If the results are acceptable, the client will be able to give the go-ahead for the next stage. A data exchange at this stage is also a requirement for UK Government projects.

The UK BIM Task Group methodologies should be followed. In particular, projects should be structured around PAS 1192-2: 2013 and data should be organised around the common format as identified in BS 1192-4: 2014. At the time of writing, not all the methodologies are available but through reference to the UK BIM Task Group's website these will be available as soon as they are published.

### UK BIM Task Group

The UK BIM Task Group's website can be found at:
www.bim-level2.org

## Operation and maintenance

The Maintenance and Operational Strategy for the project must be reviewed at this stage, to incorporate the information generated for the Developed Design. The strategy must ensure that all activities relating to the cleaning, maintenance and operation of the completed building can be undertaken safely or with minimal risk.

Clear methodologies and information need to be prepared for those who will be undertaking these operations, preferably as diagrams and other visual information. The Project Information should, as far as possible, be developed with the design team, contractors and specialists, and organised into straightforward subject areas, such as external cleaning, internal cleaning, mechanical and electrical plant and special facilities.

### Strategy for roof cleaning

Planning how to keep an atrium roof clean is always a challenge, as most building owners do not want to see cleaning equipment on permanent view inside the building.

### Strategy for roof cleaning (*continued*)

At this stage, the design team can consider a range of options, while there is enough flexibility in the design to allow any changes needed to support the one chosen. Options could include:

- design a 'garage' to house the access equipment when not in use – this would require sufficient space to be available
- integrate 'walkways' into the roof structure, so that they do not look like cleaning access
- provide temporary access, normally in the form of a mobile platform – this would usually need to be stored away from the atrium, and would require a suitable stable floor and appropriately trained staff.

Leaving the building owner and operator to devise a method is not acceptable, and would expose the client and design team to potential liability.

### Stage 3 checklist

- Are the checklists and procedures developed for the project being used?
- Is the project delivering the client's brief? Has health and safety been considered according to the brief?
- Review the list of health and safety issues:
    - ○ What health and safety issues have been resolved?
    - ○ What issues remain, and what is the plan for their resolution?
- Are conflicts and changes being identified and clearly communicated to the client?
- Are basic decisions being recorded?

## Information Exchanges

Information Exchanges required for Stage 3 are as follows:

⏐ at stage completion: the Developed Design, including the coordinated architectural, structural and building services design and updated Cost Information
⏐ for UK Government projects: an output of Project Information is required.

## Chapter summary 3

Stage 3 is crucial for the lead designer as many of the fundamentals of the project will be set out during this period. It is vital that the focus on health and safety matters is not lost among all the other activities running through this stage.

This chapter has identified the core activities that are required to maintain the approach to health and safety established during the earlier stages. These are centred around keeping the Health and Safety Strategy up to date and in balance with the increasing amount of information and complexity in the project.

The elements that contribute to the project's increasing complexity at this stage need to be well managed and carefully thought through. The team's actions, organisation and activities needed to support the process and maintain a straightforward approach at all times have been set out. For the most common or complex areas, it is worth revisiting the design periodically, to ensure that coherent and robust considerations are in place across the project.

It is essential to ensure that the good work is supported by sensible and robust exchanges of information, and that adequate records are kept, showing the path that the design has taken. However, it is important to keep these in balance: not too much and not too little. All too often it is easy to make the mistake of just lumping everything into a file. This benefits no one.

BIM is set to revolutionise this stage of the project in particular – it might even reduce many of the actions to a simple matter of choosing the right software. But many of the benefits that BIM can bring to this area are still a little way off for most projects, which is why it is important to focus on the basics.

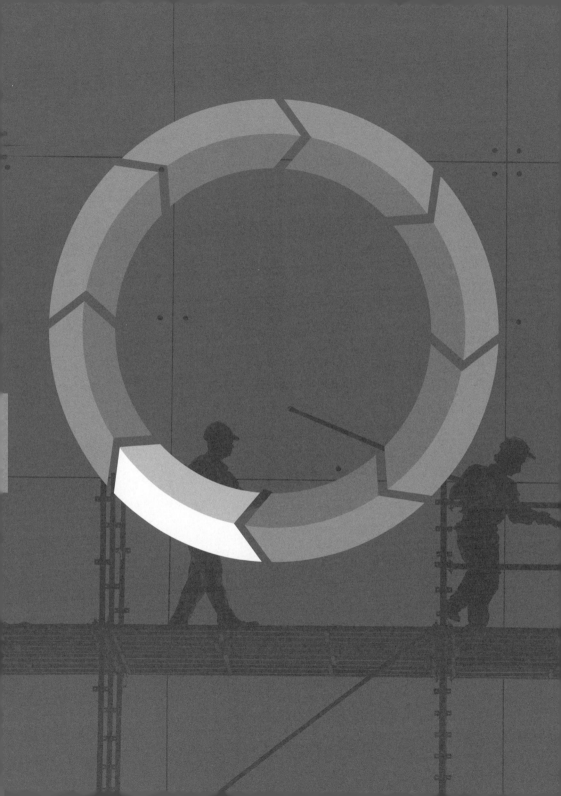

# Technical Design

# Chapter overview

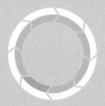

The focus at Stage 4 is on ensuring that the Technical Design meets the needs of the contractor and is developed sufficiently for the In Use stage where this is required. The Developed Design information produced in Stage 3 is now laid out in sufficient detail for the Construction stage.

The design team and contractor need to work together closely, although the procurement route will influence how this takes place, and the client needs to be kept informed. There is also dialogue with planning authorities in order to potentially close out any planning conditions, building control authorities and perhaps other third parties. A significant degree of management control is needed, to ensure the Project Strategies remain robust. Health and safety consideration must still have its place and not be sidelined by the volume of information.

The RIBA Plan of Work 2013 calls for the Technical Design to be prepared in accordance with the Project Strategies, using the core documents to ensure the team is properly organised. Here, the Design Responsibility Matrix and the working procedures established for the project should ensure that the right design team members are doing the right things. The Design Responsibility Matrix should contain both lead and supporting dutyholders for all the main areas of responsibility, so that there is an owner for each design element of health and safety focus. This should avoid any uncertainty as to who needs to ensure that a particular area has been addressed.

A large range of specialists (eg fire, accessibility, sustainability and health and safety) and informal connections (eg product systems and materials manufacturers) will be involved. Depending on the procurement route and the Building Contract selected and the Design Responsibility Matrix some Technical Design work may be undertaken by specialist subcontractors – this needs to be coordinated with the rest of the design team's work. The project's procedures must be rigorous enough to ensure that any potential risks are correctly assessed.

A degree of overlapping between Stages 4, 5 and 6 is normal, if not inevitable. Any health and safety commentary needs to reflect and allow for this.

**The key coverage in this chapter is as follows:**

Updating Project Strategies

Approach to Health and Safety Strategy

Formal information

Preparation for construction

Finalising the pre-construction information

Information Exchanges

# Introduction

The Technical Design stage of the project is when the information needed for construction becomes crystallised. It is essential that the technical analysis and verification for elements of the design are clearly included in the project documents. This stage is about getting the detail right.

Work within the project team should be progressing in accordance with the Project Strategies and Design Responsibility Matrix and following the Design Programme.

The Building Regulations submission will need to be made at this stage as the supporting technical information will now be fixed. Depending on the type of Building Contract being used, the costs and possibly the contractor will be determined during this stage. All of this requires that the Health and Safety Strategy and Project Execution Plan (including the construction phase plan and health and safety file required by the CDM regulations) are kept up to date and that any areas of uncertainty or identified hazard are examined and improved or suitable methodologies and explanations readied for the contractor.

At the end of this stage, all of the products, processes and construction principles must be identified, well understood and clearly explained. It is essential that the output is robust and coherent. It needs to be fully checked, preferably by someone from outside the design team. Those immersed within the project can overlook quite obvious issues and, especially where health and safety is concerned, become convinced everything is covered. Timing is critical here, but the need for information to be correct is paramount.

*From Stage 3*

It is important to take full advantage of the Stage 3 preparations:

Ensure the client's aspirations are still at the core of the project.

Ensure the team understands the Health and Safety Strategy.

As technical detail increases, keep focused on the potential for increased risk.

Technical approvals need to be completed to avoid potential risks later.

Use the Stage 3 format for information to make this stage easier.

## What are the Core Objectives of this stage?

The Core Objectives of the RIBA Plan of Work 2013 at Stage 4 are:

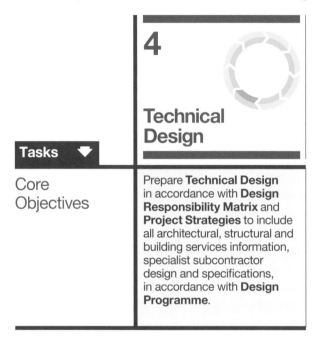

| Tasks ⬇ | **4** **Technical Design** |
|---|---|
| Core Objectives | Prepare **Technical Design** in accordance with **Design Responsibility Matrix** and **Project Strategies** to include all architectural, structural and building services information, specialist subcontractor design and specifications, in accordance with **Design Programme**. |

The Core Objectives relate to the final issue of the Technical Design, which will include all the information required for the Construction stage. The key Project Strategies need to be reviewed and updated to ensure the Technical Design follows the Final Project Brief. All the design information for architecture, structure, building services and specialist items needs to be checked and updated. Updates on regulatory compliance, contractor appointments and any other statutory actions need to be completed through a comprehensive review process.

## Updating Project Strategies

It is important that the Project Strategies are reviewed and updated during this stage, based on progress made to date. This should include the Project Execution Plan and the Construction Strategy. The latter will contain some sequencing detail that needs to be looked at carefully to tease out any risk-generating operations. This is where prior consultation with a contractor can help. The design team should have sketches of areas where complex operations are envisaged. On BIM projects, the ability to run the construction sequence (4D) is one of the greatest technical advances for safer construction. Ensure that the Project Strategies and their supporting principles are still valid and are driving the project in the right direction.

At the start of this stage, the core principles and activities of each Project Strategy should be reviewed with the client. Each of these will have a health and safety thread, so making sure they are still intact and relevant to the project detail is essential. As the design detail becomes more complex, there is increased potential for unmanaged risk.

### Project brief

The Final Project Brief will have been frozen at Stage 2. At this stage, check that the evolving technical details are consistent with the key objectives and outcomes.

### Sustainability Strategy

Balancing Sustainability Aspirations with the building's attributes, materials, equipment, etc can require some unique design solutions. Therefore, careful review of the design is required to ensure levels of risk to constructors or occupants are not raised. Use of unusual components or equipment that is not in common use, such as high-level energy collectors, wind generators or underground storage tanks, can give rise to unfamiliar risks.

### Cost Information

Cost control is now at its most sensitive. Make sure that health and safety does not suffer as a consequence of cost-reduction or value engineering measures.

### Construction Programme

As the Construction Programme (and related construction phase plan) is developed, it is likely that pressure to constrain site operations will increase. The Construction Programme must be reviewed to ensure the focus on safe operations has been maintained. Watch out for any proposed short cuts or reductions in quality or scope – they all have an effect on the potential risk. The CDM regulations require the design team to consider site-wide issues as early as possible.

### Quality

Quality, like time and cost, comes under increased pressure at this stage. Reductions in quality and performance specifications are potential triggers for a reduction in health and safety standards.

#### Quality and safety

There is clear evidence that quality and good health and safety practice are two sides of the same coin. For example, forcing brickwork to advance at too fast a rate is both unsafe and reduces quality significantly.

### Health and Safety Strategy

When reviewing the Health and Safety Strategy, continue to check that the actions it requires are proportionate with the complexity of the project. A balance is needed.

## Approach to Health and Safety Strategy

Ensure that the Technical Design is suitable for the construction phase of the project. In particular, the structure of the Health and Safety Strategy should fit logically with the rest of the technical design to be issued for construction

Consider including provisions for:

I   a project-wide health and safety communication channel
I   incentives for exemplar behaviour

| occupational health interventions, including resident on-site facilities during construction.

These are all tried-and-tested approaches.

All of the details and refinements of the design principles should be checked to ensure that they will work as intended. Each element of the building, from the largest to the smallest, needs to be identified and coordinated with its surrounding components.

Checks for regulatory compliance, required performance compliance, technical appropriateness, required aesthetics and buildability also need to be made. When undertaking these checks, every team member must aim to ensure the design is as risk-free as possible: that the architecture, structure and services will all work together, and safely.

Look for any issues that will cause hazards during construction, cleaning, maintenance or in-use activities. Some elements might have to be redesigned if they prove to be impossible, impractical or deviate from the brief. Others might require some additional consideration, perhaps due to their impact on other elements of the project, or to a lack of previous experience in their use. Examples of this kind of circumstance include the following:

| Designing very large components into the project can reduce operations on site, but they will need a skilled and trained team.
| The health and safety profiles of new materials may not be well understood by site operatives. For instance, aerogels can penetrate the skin. If their use is necessary, training and possibly specialist equipment may be needed.
| High-tolerance materials require extra time to install and possibly specialist equipment. Both requirements can draw attention away from other issues, leaving workers exposed to what would otherwise be controlled issues. For example, ensuring precast concrete components are correctly seated can expose workers to hazardous unprotected edges.
| Complex structural solutions can leave workers dealing with an unknown set of circumstances. For example, the structural engineer may be the only party with clear understanding of the erection and lifting sequence, exposing site operatives to excessive risks.
| Work at extreme height or depth, which often cannot be avoided, needs to be undertaken by those trained and experienced in such work.

## Cladding design

The cladding installation of a commercial building is one operation that needs a specialist. Cladding is often divided into separate work packages, to deliver cost and time savings. However, the lack of coordinated working means these savings may not be delivered. It also increases risk, due to the different teams working on similar areas.

In addition, the cladding specialist's recommendations for maintenance should be coordinated with other in-use considerations (eg cleaning access) to produce a design that minimises risk both during construction and when the building is occupied.

## Formal information

The project health and safety information formally required under the CDM regulations consists of the following:

I pre-construction information
I construction phase plan
I health and safety file.

### Pre-construction information

### Pre-existing information

This is a subset of the information needed to develop the project design. It will include any information about the site, including any existing structures and buildings, that may have health and safety implications.

As the information is assembled, anything that could be relevant to health and safety should be copied into a separate reference file. This will focus attention onto these elements. The file should be updated as the design progresses, and used later in assembling the health and safety file.

Any hazardous items that are identified should be assembled into a checklist or schedule, with a link to any drawn information.

## Design information (as part of the pre-construction information)

The design information must be assembled as it is developed, and formatted to make any risk management actions clear. It can be compiled from a series of templates, or as a visual risk matrix and a limited series of project documents, perhaps using marked-up drawings to identify the key issues.

The design information needs to include:

I any issues that have been considered to be important across the project from a health and safety perspective
I information covering how individual risks have been eliminated (useful if further changes occur)
I information on any remaining risks, and possible solutions for their control during site operations
I a cleaning and maintenance strategy, and detailed information on how this can be carried out with a minimum of risk
I technical information covering significant maintenance, replacement of plant etc
I information on safe demolition methodologies.

All of this information is easily assembled from the total project data. If organised well, little more than some straightforward management of files is required as the stage progresses.

### Electronic media

Using electronic media – from simple linked files and project extranets to full BIM methodologies – makes the process of managing pre-construction information much more efficient. This should not be regarded as a difficult or excessively onerous addition to the overall project demands. Clarity and organisation will make this straightforward and robust, and use of the right technology can make it an everyday process.

### Construction phase plan

At some point during Stage 4 (or in some cases earlier) the client will appoint a principal contractor. Early appointment is always recommended, as the experience and knowledge the contractor can bring to any decisions can be very helpful to the project.

Conversely, the role of principal designer may finish at the end of Stage 4, or it may continue, or continue in a limited form. If the principal designer's appointment ends, they must agree to hand over to the principal contractor all existing project information prior to work starting on site, including all of the health and safety design information and the developing health and safety file. The principal contractor will use this to produce the construction phase plan.

If the principal designer's involvement continues, they will assist with the development of the information and the analysis of further design development, which almost always occurs during Stage 5. The principal designer may be retained on a limited service to assist the principal contractor in ensuring that all the necessary design information is brought together at the end of Stage 5.

The CDM regulations require the construction phase plan to be drawn up before work starts on site. Therefore, regardless of the project team relationships, the plan is required to summarise the health and safety approach as the project nears Stage 5.

The construction phase plan must include, as a minimum:

I health and safety arrangements for the construction phase
I site rules
I special measures where work involves a particular risk (as defined in schedule 3 to the CDM regulations).

The plan needs to communicate to everyone on site what is expected, what measures and operations will be undertaken and how health and safety will be managed.

It should also:

I be relevant to the project
I clearly identify the arrangements
I be proportionate in scale and complexity to the project.

The plan should not include information that

I   is not relevant
I   masks the issues
I   comprises generic, background explanations, or
I   comprises detailed safety method statements.

## Construction phase plan contents

A typical construction phase plan will be structured as follows:

I   Description of the project, including key dates, team structure and
    Project Programme
I   Health and safety aims for the project (strategy plus developed details)
I   Site rules
I   Method for ensuring cooperation and coordination within the team
I   Arrangements for involving workers
I   Site induction procedures
I   Welfare facilities to be on site prior to construction start
I   Fire and emergency procedures for the construction phase
I   Any schedule 3 risks (mostly found in the infrastructure sector).

The content of the plan needs to be considered carefully as Stages 4
and 5 often overlap.

## The health and safety file

Prior to the 2015 revision of the CDM regulations, health and safety files
tended to include excessive information, far more than the regulations
actually required. The 2015 regulations emphasise that the file is to be
appropriate to the characteristics of the project and should contain only
relevant information (as identified below). A file is only required for projects
where there is more than one contractor.

The health and safety file must contain all the project information that
may be relevant to any subsequent work to the building. It is intended
to be used by the building's owner or operator after handover, or passed
on to any subsequent owners. It is important that the relevant technical
information is captured at this stage and included in the file. If managed
well, it can then easily be updated for handover at the end of construction.

The health and safety file will typically contain information on the following:

I Brief description of the project
I Hazards that have not been eliminated through the design or construction phases and how they have been addressed (residual risks)
I Key structural principles
I Hazardous materials used
I Removal of plant and equipment
I Health and safety for cleaning and maintenance
I Markings and identification on significant services
I As-built information, including safe access to all areas.

There needs to be enough information to identify risks, including clear information regarding any issues that have not been designed out (residual risks), but it should be in proportion to the complexity of the project. Do not include information that will not be a direct help. It can be useful to present the residual risks in a visual document, possibly as a matrix or a series of drawn and annotated illustrations, rather than a written schedule.

### Should it be in the file?

Apply the simple test:

1. Would I find the information understandable and useful?
2. Can I find the information I need easily?
3. Is anything included that is not in agreement with points 1 and 2 above.

The file should be written in a non-technical style as the owners and operators of the building might not be technically skilled in construction.

The file should have been set up, structured and developed over the course of the previous stages. With the benefit of the finalised design information, it can be developed into its final form during this stage.

### Content of the health and safety file

A quick examination will show that the required content of the health and safety file is based on and is very close to the range of information needed for the pre-construction information. Care should be taken to ensure that only relevant information is included and that pre-construction information is excluded. Relevance is the key issue: What will be directly needed by those planning and making changes in the future?

If formatted clearly, a simple edit to the relevant information at this stage will make it a straightforward operation to update and make the file ready for its final issue at Stage 6.

## Preparation for construction

During this stage the design team will be engaging with manufacturers, suppliers and specialists, who will bring to the project their assembly and construction methodologies for a range of products and materials. This will allow the team to assess the buildability of the design assumed in the Construction Strategy during Stage 2 and 3.

Ensuring the project has buildability throughout must always be a clear objective of the design team. This is as much about the information as it is about the design approach. The information needs to be presented in a manner that ensures the requirements are readily understandable; this in itself can ensure that health and safety objectives are delivered. Clarity is best achieved by using drawn information, supported where needed by appropriate specifications and supplementary data, such as test certificates or other methods of verification.

### Buildability

Buildability is the ability of the design and the specified components to come together in a practical and sensible way – one that can be readily understood by those on site. In this context, buildability is also concerned with making operations as risk free as possible.

## Considering buildability

A commonly encountered issue is the use of paints on site. Paint has been the cause of significant harm on sites in the past, and there is a new focus on the health effects of emissions from paint during application and curing.

Designers need to consider carefully the need for painted finishes. Where paints are required, the types of finish must be assessed and the appropriate products and methods specified.

An alternative solution might be to apply paint in controlled conditions off site.

The Construction Strategy needs to encompass buildability. Before the end of this stage the design team must ensure that any issues which reduce buildability have been designed out, or that special measures have been designed in to ensure they can be safely undertaken.

### Ensure safe assembly

The assembly of components on site can create many potential health and safety risks, largely because of the temporary nature of the site. The working environment is often difficult to control and conditions can change rapidly, creating an unsatisfactory workplace. Dust protection,

## Buildability issues: design out or design in

| | |
|---|---|
| Cutting of components on site | Design out |
| Oversized components | Design out |
| Excessively bulky or heavy components | Design out |
| High-level or deep workface | Special measures required |
| Repetitive operations | Design to be factory based or automate |
| Risk of dust, particles or vapour | Design out, or design in special measures |
| Sealants, glues, compounds etc | Special measures required |

control of guarding and distractions from other operations can all impact on detailed operations.

The design team need to work through the assembly patterns in the Technical Design to ensure that risks are kept to a minimum and that one safe approach is described in the documents. This is where a BIM methodology really works. As mentioned for Stage 3, the BIM model can be used to visualise the construction sequence, helping the designers and constructors to determine the safest approach.

### Information issue for construction

At the end of Stage 4, the building envelope and all external details will be fully developed and finalised. All interior details will also be finalised, if included in the contract. The services – electrical, mechanical, plumbing, fire, IT – will all be finalised.

Prescriptive products and materials will be included in the specification as descriptive and performance-based aspects are often finalised by the contractor and specialist subcontractors. The specification should also contain specific clauses relating to health and safety. As the specification is in many cases a contractual document, inclusion of such clauses can have a real effect, ensuring good outcomes by specifying low-risk options.

### The specification: health and safety clauses

Clauses that support industry health and safety initiatives can be included in the specification. While these may have limited authority, they reinforce the intention that all construction should be as safe as possible. Such clauses can be based on the 2012 Construction Commitments (currently under revision). Below are a few examples.

- Appropriate skills and experience
  All site staff shall be required to hold a Construction Skills Certification Scheme (CSCS) card.
- Manual handling
  In accordance with the Manual Handling Regulations, all components shall be installed in a manner that avoids

## The specification: health and safety clauses
(*continued*)

excessive manual loading. Attention is drawn to the HSE
guidance on manual handling and it is assumed this will be
adopted throughout the construction programme.
– Generation of dust
Airborne dust is to be avoided at all times, regardless of
the process or materials involved. Where dust generation is
unavoidable and subject to prior discussion with the design
team and client, measures must be adopted to ensure that
dust is completely contained and that all operatives wear
comprehensive PPE (personal protective equipment).
– Onsite cutting
The construction details have been developed to minimise
cutting on site. Where it is unavoidable it must be subject to
strict controls. An environment as near as possible to factory
conditions needs to be created and full PPE used by all
operatives, who are also subject to safe working patterns.
High-risk operations, such as high-level or heavy materials
cutting, must be subject to a rigorously planned work
procedure that is strictly adhered to.
– Use of materials that can cause harm
Use of materials that can cause harm has been kept to a
minimum. Where they are used, installation processes, PPE
and appropriate training must be in place. For instance, when
pouring concrete it must be done such that no operative will
have any direct skin contact with the material at any time.
Other materials that need to be controlled are lead, some
paints, glues and solvents, and composites that give off high
levels of volatile organic compounds.

As Technical Design documents are completed, nearing that point where
they are signed off 'for construction', a health and safety check should be
undertaken. This should be a separate process, which looks at all drawn,
written and third-party information solely from a risk analysis perspective.
Any observations should be recorded and included with the information
for issue. If significant issues are identified, they could require a change
to the information concerned.

Issued information must contain clear explanations of all health and
safety aspects. These do not have to be lengthy or complex, but just give
the essence of what has been done, or what needs to be done, to ensure

risk is controlled. This can be most usefully conveyed in a drawn form or as sections in specifications. Giving the pattern of this information across the whole of the project is helpful for the team, as it provides simple and clear direction. If for any reason some element is missing, it stands out.

## SHE boxes

Some projects have required information boxes on all drawings and documents (the so-called SHE box – safety, health and environment). However, these do not work as they quickly become a chore, repeating the same issues, and are largely ignored. If there are no unusual issues, or no special measures have been undertaken, then say so clearly.

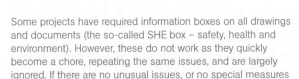

### Finalising the cleaning and maintenance strategies

The Maintenance and Operational Strategy should be checked again and updated as necessary. It needs to cover the design team's approach and the preferred methodology to all elements within the building. Clearly, some information could still change, especially if significant packages are to be designed by a specialist subcontractor, such as curtain walling when details of the walling design may not yet be known. Where possible, the design team should move from using their own information to using that provided by the actual manufacturer or supplier.

## Cleaning and maintenance schedule

This update of the cleaning and maintenance schedule should contain the following:

– An overall description of the project
– Key contact information
– A site layout, including all significant features
– Details of all elevations and the roof
– Principles of external cleaning and maintenance
– A schedule of all internal finishes and cleaning processes
– An explanation of any difficult areas, such as atria ceilings

### Cleaning and maintenance schedule (*continued*)

– Any other health and safety relevant information, such as proximity to natural hazards, eg rivers, cliffs, existing buildings or industrial complexes.

This will form the basis of the final document, which can be easily completed towards the end of Stage 5, when all equipment and component details have been defined.

### Regulatory verification

Checking that the Technical Design complies with health and safety legislation is obviously an important requirement. However, verification that the design complies with town planning and Building Regulations requirements is also relevant to health and safety. If the design does not comply with these requirements, late changes to the design may be required.

Late changes are always risky as they can never be as well considered as the other design details. Compromises may have to be made, due to the inevitable time and cost constraints, potentially adding new risks to the design.

### Change Control Procedures

As the Technical Design is signed off and contracts with the supply chain and possibly contractors are agreed, technical details become expensive and complex to change.

To ensure best practice over change control, the Change Control Procedures established in earlier stages (see page 123: Stage 3) must continue to be applied rigidly.

## Finalising the pre-construction information

The CDM regulations require that the construction team is in possession of all relevant information prior to work starting on site. Towards the end of this stage, it is important that a complete review of this information is undertaken.

The pre-construction information should be assessed against the following characteristics:

| Appropriate
   Only information that is relevant to the project should be included – this is especially true for the health and safety information. Anything else diverts attention and may lead to important issues being overlooked.

| Good quality
   Information must be of the best quality achievable. It must be clear and concise, the content well organised and the object apparent.

| Organised
   The project information as a whole needs to be ordered. It should ideally be structured according to an acknowledged referencing system. It should have an index identifying the current and future information, allowing for changes and expansion. The overall project should be broken down logically, and then each section further divided to make identification of finite areas very straightforward. All health and safety information needs to be clearly highlighted. Individual documents, drawings and electronic files also need this level of care and attention, with an organised layout and referencing system throughout.

| Verified
   As far as possible, every piece of information should be verified and that verification held on record. It is rare that this is needed, but as a principle of good practice it builds confidence in the issued information.

| Coordinated
   A watchword of the whole CDM process, this is also a mainstream design objective. All the information issued needs to agree across every parameter. The checking process prior to issue for construction must consider every part of the project information set and ensure that it all ties up.

| Agreed
   In the process of checking and verification, making sure the information has been agreed by the client, their representatives, the planning authority, the building control body, relevant statutory authorities, significant suppliers and the design team is fundamental.

I Complete

Before issue, check that all the information is available and that every point has been covered. Sometimes it is not possible for the information to be complete due to the timing of procurement or ongoing design development. It is helpful if the issued information identifies where these additional areas are and broadly what can be expected.

## Procurement

It is particularly important at this stage to keep under review any changes that occur due to procurement decisions. Under some Building Contract forms the contractor may choose to procure entirely different products or assemblies from those originally identified. This can reintroduce a risk that has previously been designed out, change a risk that has been identified and explained in the pre-construction information, or reduce the risk profile. The risk implications of any such changes need to be confirmed for all significant design elements. This will require a thorough understanding of the risks, and a full discussion with the contractor and client before final orders are placed.

## Information Exchanges

Information Exchanges required for Stage 4 are as follows:

I at stage completion: the completed Technical Design for the project
I for UK Government projects: not required.

## Chapter summary 4

Stage 4 is a complex stage. With many activities occurring simultaneously, it needs good management and careful preparation. Providing the right information to the right people at the right time has never been so important as during this stage.

This stage requires the Technical Design detail to be developed, the Information Exchange to be assembled, perhaps in packages, and the final checks to be carried out prior to construction. When under pressure to get the information out to the contractor, it is all too easy to lose focus on health and safety risk management.

This chapter has identified the structure of the pre-construction information and the health and safety file and some of the shortcuts available for their preparation.

The Technical Design process will often involve specialist subcontractors. Design work undertaken outside of the design team – whether for large elements, such as cladding, or small assemblies – needs to be managed with equal care.

Ensuring that the Technical Design covers all aspects of construction before work starts on site is always the right and most rewarding approach.

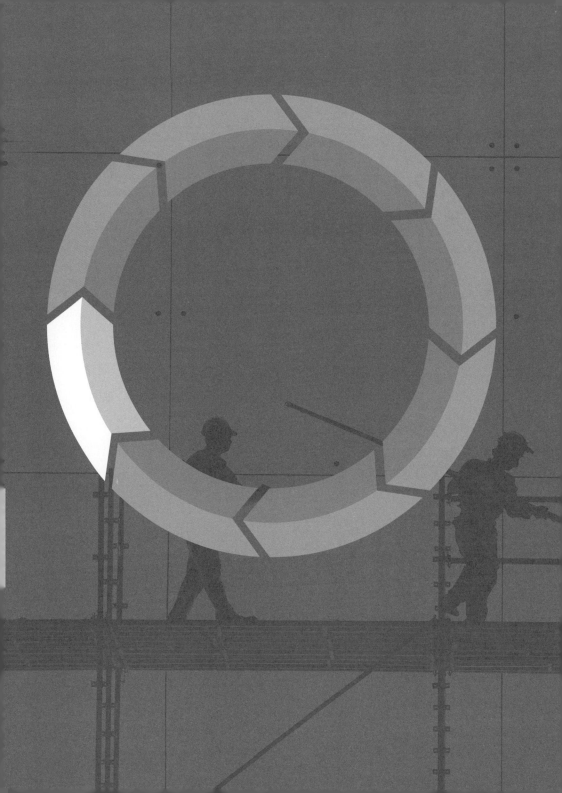

# Construction

# Chapter overview

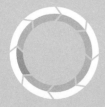

In this stage the project moves to site. The bulk of the design work will have been completed before the start of construction, although with many forms of procurement Stages 4 and 5 will overlap, as set out in the Project Programme. On most projects some additional design will be required as construction progresses, in response to Design Queries – those in authority at this stage need to be alert to any CDM issues that may arise as a result.

There will be construction and assembly activities taking place both on and off site, therefore significant management skill will be needed. Many projects fall behind at this point due to lack of control across the different areas, mostly due to poor or uncoordinated information. The RIBA Plan of Work 2013 focuses on the control of the project, ensuring that the Project Strategies are maintained.

A large number of operations will be required to ensure a smooth transition to activity on site. Elements and assemblies may have to be manufactured off site or products bought in from a wide range of sources. Manufacturing of key components should have been under way for some time, especially for items with long lead times, and materials may have to have been pre-ordered to avoid delays in site progress.

The management focus will be on the Construction Programme and the interaction between the contractor and specialist suppliers. The former should be reinforcing the Project Objectives and updating the key Project Strategies, such as the Sustainability Strategy, the Health and Safety Strategy and the Handover Strategy.

A series of meetings and Information Exchanges are needed to ensure everyone in the project team has the correct information at the right time.

Often, the construction sequences will be modified from those previously planned, perhaps due to unforeseen issues on site, planning constraints or manufacturing difficulties. This may require changes to be made to the design information at a time when there is great pressure to ensure timely delivery. Keeping control of possible hazards during this phase can be extremely challenging.

**The key coverage in this chapter is as follows:**

Pre-construction actions

Changes and substitutions

The construction phase plan

On-site progress

Updating the health and safety file

Review of the works

Nearing completion

Handover information

Information Exchanges

# Introduction

As start on site approaches, the contractor needs to review all the information and satisfy themselves that it is complete and gives a clear understanding of the project, particularly of the risks involved. It is crucial that there will be sufficient and continuous communication within the project team on site, and that processes for resolving Design Queries are in place. These need to be handled by the design team with the same care and attention as the previously issued design information.

Making sure all the issues are covered from a health and safety perspective can be challenging, especially on a complex or fast-moving project. Using your systems and procedures can make this straightforward and ensure that vital issues are not missed.

Making sure the 'As-constructed' Information is complete for handover is also a key challenge at this time. Cooperation within the project team is necessary for this to be effective. The responsibility for ensuring 'As-constructed' Information is produced can vary from project to project. This should have been agreed with the client from the start, as part of the Handover Strategy. In some situations – where there is an emphasis on specialist subcontractor design – the exact detail of what has been constructed and installed might only be known by a few members of the on-site team. Whoever has the responsibility to record this information needs to maintain good communication with those team members. It is essential that the 'As-constructed' Information is accurate.

The Project Strategies should ensure that accurate 'As-constructed' Information is gathered for both the general records and the health and safety file.

*From Stage 4*

It is important to take full advantage of the Stage 4 preparations:

Ensure there is a full review with the client and contractor.

Review the information issued for construction.

Ensure the construction phase information and plan are in place.

Check all items where risk remains.

Check changes caused by procurement.

Summarise the health and safety position across the project.

Update information for the health and safety file.

## What are the Core Objectives of this stage?

The Core Objectives of the RIBA Plan of Work 2013 at Stage 5 are:

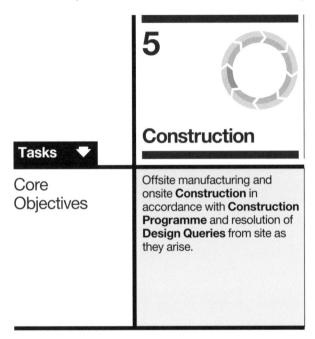

The Core Objectives of the plan of work at this stage revolve around ensuring that construction goes according to plan. A key element of this is to ensure that any Design Queries raised by the contractor are brought to a close.

### Implications of the Building Contract

The Building Contract between the client and the contractor for the construction of the project needs to be understood by the design team. Depending on the Design Responsibility Matrix incorporated into the Building Contract, specialist subcontractors may be required to provide design services during Stage 4. This design work still needs the same level of risk assessment and management.

On certain projects, more than one Building Contract may be required; for example, one for shell and core works and another for interiors, furniture, fittings and equipment. These may also include regular site inspections and review of progress.

The procurement route may also dictate the Project Programme and may result in certain stages overlapping or being undertaken concurrently.

## Pre-construction actions

The project set-up should have been made clear at Stage 1, in the Contractual Tree and Design Responsibility Matrix, among other key documents. The areas of authority, responsibility and arrangements for control and issue of information – both prior to and during the on-site stage – will vary considerably, but should all be clear. At the start of Stage 5 it is essential that all of these are revisited and checked with the client and the contractor's team.

The agreed procedures must also be checked, to ensure they are still relevant and will be implemented by everyone involved across the project. It is common for changes in personnel, especially in the client's team, to necessitate changes to procedures. If such changes are required, there must be agreement on how any new procedures will work.

## Exemplar industry health and safety actions

A range of exemplar schemes can be implemented to encourage and support good health and safety on site (normally instigated by the client):

- social media health and safety project channel
- reward schemes for exemplary behaviour
- bonding schemes, such as 'Don't Walk By'
- national schemes with a health and safety requirement, such as the Considerate Constructors Scheme
- occupational health specialists for the project.

### Liaison within the project team

### Information and processes

There are several overlapping actions that need to take place to ensure the overall progress of the project and, in particular, that all health and safety actions progress smoothly to site.

I Checking of design information, to ensure it contains full explanations of the health and safety considerations and objectives.
I Carrying out ongoing design (depending on the procurement route), which may be happening in many locations.
I Ensuring the principal contractor has sufficient information to produce the construction phase plan before starting on site.
I Ensuring that town planning conditions have been discharged, where possible. Often, some will require verification through the procurement process or for site progress
I Checking that, as far as possible, all Building Regulations matters have been signed off. As with planning conditions, some can only be signed off once progress has been made.

It is important to ensure that no overlooked errors remain in the Project Information, to avoid any last-minute changes.

## Responsibilities and roles

During the lead up to starting on site, the emphasis needs to move from the design team to the contractor. The design team will have largely concluded their activities, but the contractor will be mobilising their team, including members from the supply chain. It is critical that the health and safety information is transferred smoothly, to ensure the objectives are properly conveyed.

The exact roles and their responsibilities at this time will vary depending on the contract and appointments. Significantly, the CDM 2015 regulations allow for a number of options. The principal designer role may continue throughout the construction phase. In this case, the same broad responsibilities apply: all design issues should be reviewed for risk, and any that are identified must be minimised or controlled. However, overall responsibility for matters relating to health and safety on site is transferred to the principal contractor.

The principal contractor and the core construction team will ideally have been appointed some time before work starts on site, to allow adequate time for mobilisation. During this period the construction phase plan can be prepared, taking into account the design team's information, when any further design development is needed and the impact of any regulatory requirements not yet signed off.

There is also the possibility that the principal designer role may finish at the point when site operations are started, in which case the principal contractor needs to take over their duties.

### Control of information

Regular structured, formal meetings are still necessary for projects on site. The design team must continue to be represented and the appropriate degree of health and safety information discussed.

Many teams and clients insist that health and safety is the first item on the agenda of all formal meetings. This is good practice, as long as the issues are properly discussed. It is also important to structure the reporting at these meetings in a consistent and logical manner, so that issues are not overlooked.

Good communication outside meetings is also essential. The aim should be to cultivate an atmosphere that encourages the design team and the construction team to help each other. In the competitive and commercially driven construction industry, this is not always easy to achieve, but it should be a critical project objective.

Informal health and safety focus meetings can also contribute to this goal. Designers should attend on-site briefings, inductions and specialist meetings, so they gain a greater understanding of the on-site operations. Equally, the construction team should be invited to attend design and development review meetings. This will encourage greater understanding and shared viewpoints. Often, where problems do emerge it is because the design and construction teams do not share the same perspective or are not aware of each other's point of view.

It is essential for the development of better health and safety that everyone in the project team has as wide an understanding as possible, so that when issues surface, everyone can contribute to the development of the solution.

### Sharing information

Good team communication relies on high-quality information. When preparing information to be shared, ask yourself the following:

- Does it say what it is? The introduction and title need to be clear and obvious.
- Does it say who produced it and why?
- Is it clear, organised and in a commonly understandable format?
- Is it understandable by the intended audience?
- Is it relevant and logical?
- Is it version controlled? If further versions are required, is this clearly identified?

## Changes and substitutions

Design changes during construction can be required for a number of reasons, the most obvious being cost or time overruns, due to errors coming to light or because earlier assumptions were incorrect. To some degree, these can be avoided by taking proper care in the earlier stages – during Stages 2 and 3 – to set the right path for design development, and to ensure that the work consolidated in Stage 4 is robust and coherent. On larger projects, with complex supply chains and long lead-in times, later operations often have to make last-minute changes in order to correct for these mistakes. However, the final design must be comprehensive and buildable.

Often, however, the design information has not been fully coordinated in every detail, which creates conflicts of time, money and practicalities. The construction team might have an opinion on how to deal with these conflicts, and a client faced with their arguments will clearly accept the degree of certainty they offer. However, such changes can often lead to very poor outcomes. One of these might be a change to the risk profile that the design team have developed for a particular element. It is essential that the design team keep ahead of this situation. They must be able to justify the design and its implications. They must also be able to review issues with the construction team and come up with a consistent health and safety solution.

### How to manage change during construction

Any changes to the design after Stage 2 should follow the Change Control Procedures established for the project (see page 123: Stage 3). Therefore any design changes made after work starts on site must also follow these procedures.

Any change control documentation should clearly show:

I  what has been undertaken to minimise risk, during a change
I  what still needs to be done to minimise risk, as a response to a change.

If this approach is adopted at the start, when information is handed over to the contractor, changes can be highlighted and checked against potential risks and, if necessary, flagged for review. The review decides if the change adds risk or not: if it does, it needs to be reconsidered until it is either removed or is manageable.

## The construction phase plan

The construction phase plan, a requirement of the CDM regulations, must be ready to implement before work starts on site, for use as the controlling mechanism from that point. It should be started as early as possible, and certainly as soon as the principal contractor is appointed.

Each of the dutyholders has a part to play in the preparation of the plan:

| The client must ensure it is drawn up prior to the start of construction works.
| The principal contractor must draw up the plan based on the information provided by the team through the principal designer (comprising pre-project information, project information and any further information arising from the pre-start liaison between the design team and the construction team).
| The principal designer has a duty to help the principal contractor create and develop the plan.

Once generated, the principal contractor then needs to keep the plan up to date and ensure it reflects any further changes on the project.

The critical issue throughout the construction phase is that it is regarded as a live document. It should be used as a regular reference, and therefore the requirement to keep it updated and current becomes part of the normal working pattern.

## On-site progress

For most projects, a competent contractor given adequate and comprehensive information will formulate a plan and manage the health and safety risks accordingly. However, there will often be occasions when the design team will be required to provide additional input, perhaps to provide clarification on specific details or to assess the full implications of a change to the design. The design team should always be aware of progress and of any issues that have developed on site so that they can assist effectively.

## Problems on site

A range of unforeseen issues can arise on site with the potential to disrupt progress.

I Underground issues
Undetected below-ground issues could include:
  o geological problems (eg soft spots)
  o unrecorded disused services
  o old mine workings
  o flooding cause by underground streams.

I Materials shortages
Short-term or unexpected materials shortages can result in last-minute changes, affecting the risk profile. The changed risks need to be assessed and managed.

I Information
Even where every effort is made to ensure issued information is correct, errors can occur. While BIM will vastly improve this situation, it is critical to ensure that everyone is working to the correct information.

I Third party problems
Projects can be subject to third party problems, such as industrial strikes, transportation problems, fires nearby, most of which cannot be foreseen and will cause problems on site. These need the whole team to review the implications.

Contractors will often have fully developed contingency plans and policies for dealing with such issues. Having these in place will reduce reaction times and minimise the potential risks.

## Considerate Constructors Scheme

Many contractors belong to the Considerate Constructors Scheme. A nationwide scheme, it requires contractors to have a well-organised and proactive approach to all of their projects. It particularly emphasises the need for measures to control the impact the project may have on neighbouring communities and individuals. It is seen as a mark of good practice and well-managed health and safety.

## Updating the health and safety file

Throughout this stage, the health and safety file should be updated by the principal designer or principal contractor in preparation for handover to the client at Stage 6.

There are always changes and updates to information during the construction phase. The file needs to reflect the information current at this time. As covered in Stage 4 (page 149), the health and safety file must be proportionate to the project; there has been a tendency in the past to include an excess of detail, making the information handed over almost useless.

### Keep it brief

Keeping it brief but relevant and useful can be a challenge. It is useful to organise information in the health and safety file on the basis of how frequently it is likely to be used: immediately, weekly, monthly, annually, in a few years' time and, finally, decades in the future. Of course, information can be cross-referenced for ease of use.

### Start the health and safety file early

This stage in the project will be highly demanding for everyone. It is therefore much better to have developed the health and safety file gradually, rather than to attempt to assemble it now. The file structure and most of the contents can be prepared beforehand, requiring only minimal work to complete it after construction ends.

## Review of the works

In the days and weeks before Handover, a thorough review of the project will be required. Depending on the contractual responsibilities, this could be undertaken by one of the project team members or all of them. Some teams conduct a detailed checking process, traditionally called 'snagging'.

Commissioning of the main services systems, if present, will also be undertaken during this period. It is essential that the focus on the health and safety threads of the project is retained. This stage involves many systems coming together for the first time. It is essential that the safety-critical items are carefully checked and that any issues are identified for remedy.

The focus should be on:

I   services and plant operation
I   access and maintenance provisions
I   fire safety systems
I   information on safe operation
I   completion, testing and commissioning of these systems.

Remember that regulation 38(2) of the Building Regulations 2010 requires a complete explanation of the fire strategy and any fire safety-related systems to be provided. This needs to be approved by the building control body before they are able to sign off the Building Regulations application. This is normally the responsibility of the design team.

## Nearing completion

The lead-up to Practical Completion is a critical time in any project. Time and resources can become stretched, no matter how well organised the project is, and there is always a risk that health and safety issues could be overlooked.

Good close teamwork is required. To help the project team with the final preparations before handover:

I   make sure that all the key points are flagged up and, if necessary, initiate special briefings
I   give everyone a 'pep talk' and encourage them to revisit everything they have been doing
I   use pre-prepared checklists to ensure everything is completed.

As all the design elements finally come together, the contractor may well need help to interpret some issues. Planning and Building Regulations completion and sign-off should also be achieved at this time.

## Handover information

The Handover Strategy (drawn up at Stage 1 and updated during the design stages) should define the process for this part of the project, based on the size of the project and the procurement route selected. The aim should be to provide as much clearly organised, relevant and accurate information as possible to the client, as close to the Practical Completion date as possible.

The requirements of the CDM regulations will be met by the handover of the health and safety file (see above).

### 'As-constructed' Information

Compilation of 'As-constructed' Information is essential. Information issued at handover is often based on the design team's 'final construction issue' information, and so does not capture any deviations between the design and what was actually built. It is therefore important the 'As-constructed' Information is compiled and updated continuously throughout the Construction stage. The 'As-constructed' Information also needs to include 'as-built' information from any specialist subcontractors. It is essential that the recorded information is as accurate as possible, ensuring that the operator of the building will use the design team's prescribed methods and safest approaches.

A detailed plan for preparing information for handover to the client should emerge from the Handover Strategy and be implemented in good time. This should include key milestones for information production.

### BIM model

The use of BIM offers huge advantages over conventional methods. In particular, a BIM model of the as-constructed building can be used by the owner's facilities management team during the In Use phase. The BIM model identifies exactly what has been used in the building, how it all works together and exact product details, and so could be used to monitor and check performance and identify maintenance processes.

## Information Exchanges

Information Exchanges required for Stage 5 are as follows:

I   at stage completion: 'As-constructed' Information
I   for UK Government projects: not required.

| **Chapter summary** | 5 |
|---|---|

The construction phase is the culmination of months of planning, preparation and hard work. It is critical that the team ensures the correct approach to health and safety is adopted on site. The Health and Safety Strategy may include the construction team implementing additional measures, perhaps joining the Considerate Constructors Scheme or other industry initiatives.

The contractor should check the information given to them thoroughly for issues that may increase risk to those on site. The procurement route will fundamentally affect roles and responsibilities and how information is exchanged during this stage – the appropriate procedures and strategies must have been put in place prior to work starting on site. The design team also need to ensure that any changes made to the design during construction impose no greater level of risk.

At the end of the construction phase, it is essential that the 'As-constructed' Information and other items required at handover are collated and that all outstanding conditions and sign-offs have been completed. Good organisation, communication and team working is critical at this stage.

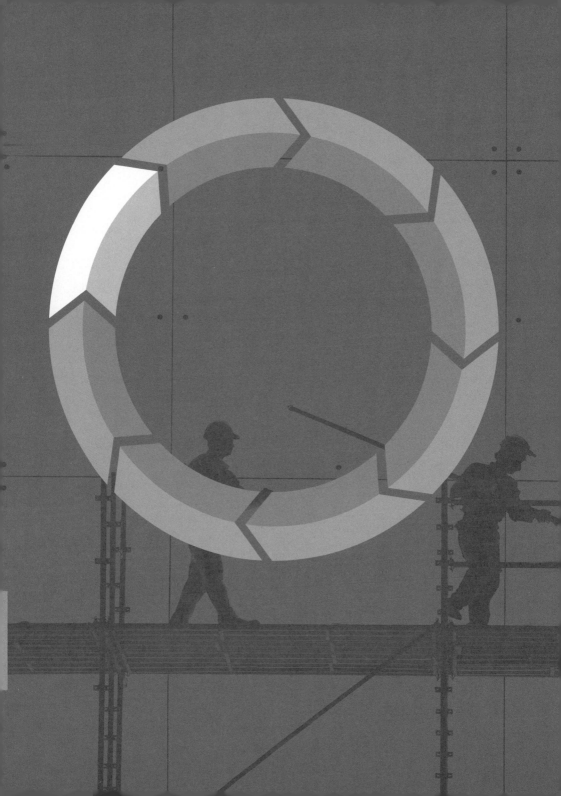

# Handover and Close Out

# Chapter overview

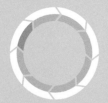

The RIBA Plan of Work 2013 makes it very clear that careful attention needs to be given to the handover of the project. The Handover Strategy needs to be planned from the start and developed as the project progresses to ensure there is a well-organised and properly planned handover.

While processes for organised handover have been available for many years, there has been reticence to develop them and use them to their full potential. Formalised handover techniques have been used in the public sector to good effect, and larger clients have also driven this approach. While these have concentrated on building performance primarily from an environmental perspective, there is clearly equal benefit for health and safety too.

For projects in the mainstream there is the issue of cost – Who pays for the additional resources needed? – and some concerns over liability if faults are found. There is no doubt that to implement a good handover process and apply proper management at this stage will cost more than simply adopting the 'finish and forget' approach often seen.

For the project to be properly finished, delivered and operating as designed, there needs to be a clear and organised completion, with the whole project team involved. The provision of clear information at handover is essential, especially for operational matters. The owners and users of the building must be involved in this process, to ensure they thoroughly understand their facility.

Increasingly, clients require buildings to perform as designed. Therefore, a system for measuring the performance of the building in operation has to be part of delivery. The issue of liability if performance is not as designed is complex and of concern to many designers. Until better and more accurate delivery and verification is commonplace, the legal issues around this subject will remain unresolved.

However, the increasing digitalisation of the construction industry is bringing with it reliable data, enabling construction based on robust information and allowing systems to be fully tested in the virtual world, prior to handover. This brings new hope that, in future, close out and handover will mean something reliable and positive. Structured information exchanges, as required in government projects, will also aid this outcome.

UK Government projects may require an Information Exchange if BIM is being used.

**The key coverage in this chapter is as follows:**

The handover

Health and safety at handover

Close out tasks

Operation and maintenance information

Soft Landings

Review of Project Performance

Project Information update

Information Exchanges

# Introduction

At this stage, the Handover Strategy needs to be applied thoroughly.

The handover process needs to take owners and occupiers through the complete range of issues and information pertaining to the completed building. It is important to recognise that the team will have been working on the project for a considerable time, in some cases years, and so may easily overlook obvious issues or not realise that details they take for granted might not be readily understandable by other people.

It is also important to take full advantage of the Stage 5 preparations.

Review the handover information for completeness and quality.

Ensure the client's aspirations have been achieved.

Make sure there is still a focus on health and safety.

Ensure any changes are included in the 'As-constructed' Information.

## What are the Core Objectives of this stage?

The Core Objectives of the RIBA Plan of Work 2013 at Stage 6 are:

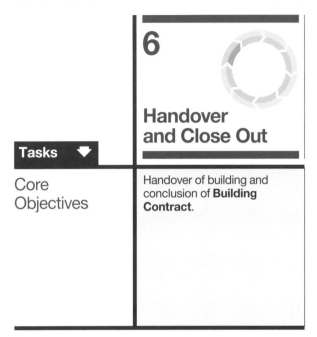

The Core Objectives at this stage require that the Handover Strategy is applied in full. The Project Information must be given to the building's owner and occupier in a managed and controlled manner, and the close out of items must ensure that any remaining risks are properly controlled.

Any Post-occupancy Evaluation processes are set up at this point, so that Feedback can be generated for the benefit of any future projects.

## The handover

Handover can be stressful. There always seem to be issues that crop up at the last minute, demanding time and resources to resolve. It is therefore essential that everything that can be prepared in advance has been prepared. The structure of the RIBA Plan of Work 2013 encourages and supports this approach.

All paperwork that can be prepared in advance should be drawn up, checked and made ready, particularly test certificates, verification information, formal approvals, materials checklists and record data. All of these will have an element of health and safety, even if not immediately obvious.

### Before handover

In the run up to handover, a number of things must have been agreed by the project team:

I the timetable for handover
I who will be involved in undertaking what actions
I what sign-offs are needed, who will give them and how they will be recorded
I what happens if things go wrong, ie put an agreed plan B in place
I who needs to be informed of what – perhaps not all information is needed by everyone.

### Check and review

Before handover takes place, take a step back and ensure that all elements of the Handover Strategy are covered.

After handover, take time to look back and review and reflect on all the actions taken. Hold debriefs with the design team and, preferably, the whole project team. Above all, look at the lessons learned and capture the important points in a file for use at Stage 0 of the next project.

## Health and safety at handover

At this stage, health and safety activities mainly relate to the handing over of information to the building's users and owners. For the most part, the information will have been prepared as part of the ongoing design process. Therefore, apart from ensuring it is up to date, there should be no need to produce health and safety information exclusively for this stage.

The information to be handed over needs to be logical and clear and prepared to a high professional standard, and should cover the following issues:

| The health and safety file
The health and safety file should be virtually complete and taking key contacts through its contents should be a high priority. The core information in the file will give most of the information needed by owners and occupants (see page 149: Stage 4 for details of the contents), including clear information regarding any issues that have not been designed out (residual risks).

| Emergency information
The fire and emergency procedures.

| Regulations and compliance
Any information required to comply with the CDM regulations, town planning and Building Regulations.

| Cleaning and maintenance
The general access, cleaning and maintenance provisions, clearly laid out in a separate document.

| Building facilities and characteristics
The overall building design, facilities and general construction principles. This should also identify any unusual issues in respect of demolition, or that need to be considered if alterations are carried out in the future.

Also helpful is an explanation of all the information sources and where to find specific points. The use of digital data and BIM methodologies will create opportunities for this information to be more easily accessible and allow a variety of formats to be used.

### The workplace regulations

Under the workplace regulations and CDM regulations, there are two critical considerations to be addressed at handover. The design team, especially the principal designer, need to:

I review the completed building and ensure that, so far as is reasonably practicable, all aspects of the regulations have been addressed, and
I ensure that the building's owners and occupiers are aware of their responsibilities under the workplace regulations.

## Close out tasks

As part of the Handover Strategy, the closing out tasks need to be undertaken in a managed and logical format. There are key areas that need to be sequenced and addressed as the project nears handover. Activities that can involve a high degree of risk include:

I site security
I traffic management
I high-level cleaning and commissioning
I removal of temporary structures, services or plant
I transfer from construction safety systems to permanent systems, eg fire alarm
I ownership, authority and insurance verifications.

### Handover inspection

For many projects it will be necessary to carry out an examination of the building. The degree of involvement of the design team in this process will vary depending on the size and complexity of the project and the contract structure. For some projects, the verification of the building will rest entirely with the construction team, while on others the design team and the construction team will both be involved. In some cases, the client will also want their team to be part of the process.

Whoever is conducting the inspection, they should follow some straightforward principles:

I Everyone needs to be briefed on the health and safety aspects of the building, almost as if going to site for the first time. While being readied for handover, there may still be areas that are incomplete, being commissioned or in final cleaning, all of which may be hazardous.
I Everyone should approach the inspection with the normal rules of site visits uppermost in their minds. While the building may look complete, it might not be safe. The construction team must advise on remaining

hazards and safeguards, such as the need to wear personal protection equipment (PPE).

| Team members may choose to wear PPE in any event, certainly at the start this is always a good idea.

| Everyone should receive the same information and briefing as to the required complete state and performance. They should be on the lookout for any variance from the requirements.

| Obviously significant issues need to be addressed immediately, and with others a proportionate approach needs to be taken. A 'personal safety first' approach is necessary at all times.

| Reports of any issues must be included within the general reporting. Depending on the seriousness of the issues discovered, they may need to be put right prior to handover. Others may be addressed later.

## Completeness at handover

There are always some elements that are difficult to close out prior to handover. The Handover Strategy should define exactly what will be fully complete and what will not. Sometimes, systems will need fine tuning, which can only be done during occupation. The aim should be to ensure that as much of the project as possible is fully complete and working. This in itself may give rise to hazards that have to be controlled. For example, will the building's final cleaning system be used for the pre-handover clean? If not, what temporary provisions are in place and are they safe?

## 'As-constructed' Information

The 'As-constructed' Information must continue to be updated during this stage, to ensure it properly represents the building as it was when finally handed over. It will comprise a mixture of 'as-built' information from specialist subcontractors and the 'final construction issue' information from design team members. The client may also wish to undertake an 'as-built' survey at this stage, using new surveying technologies to bring a further degree of accuracy to this information.

Some of the information will be sensitive, such as details of security systems, key codes and mastering, operations of safety critical systems projects, so information security will be an important consideration.

The information should continue to be updated in response to ongoing client Feedback and maintenance or operational developments.

## Operation and maintenance information

All aspects of the completed building should be able to be operated, maintained and cleaned safely or with minimum risk. Clear guidance needs to be prepared to ensure that those taking on the 'In Use' building operations can do so safely.

All in-use activities should be covered in the operation and maintenance (O&M) information handed over at this stage. This will derive directly from the Maintenance and Operational Strategy devised initially during Stage 2: Concept Design. This information needs to be comprehensive and well organised. Increasingly, this is prepared in an electronic format, allowing easy search and smart indexing, so that information can be found quickly. It is essential this information is accurate and reflects exactly what is needed.

The information in the health and safety file should be entirely separate. However, good practice would be to include the health and safety information in the O&M manuals as well. This allows it to be seen in the context of the other in-use activities.

Developments in BIM will allow a full set of graphical digital and contract information to be handed over along with comprehensive operating guidance. This will offer the prospect of creating a fully detailed information set, usable from every perspective.

During the handover phase, clear guidance on the following areas should be provided, whether in the O&M manuals or via a programme of user training:

I External areas and features
Safe access to all areas should be identified, permitting safe operation. High-level lighting, security fences and powered gates, landscape features (especially those involving water) and retaining walls should all have well-considered, safe explanations for normal operational use and maintenance.

I External facades
The handover should include a full demonstration, or training in the case of complex systems, as set out and described in the Maintenance and Operational Strategy. The O&M manual should include full information.

| Roofs and terraces
Safe access is always needed to these areas, whether for general maintenance or for occasional repairs. The approach is the same as for facades and should be described in the O&M information.

| High-level services, signs and features
It is important that items such as these are not overlooked, and that adequate guidance is provided in the O&M manuals. A whole-team approach is needed to ensure that all situations have been covered. Commonly overlooked elements include aerials, sensors and lightning protection systems.

| Internal high-level areas
Any high-level interior areas need to have their own cleaning and maintenance systems. These need to be fully demonstrated during handover.

| Internal cleaning
Internal cleaning and maintenance systems need to be fully itemised in the documentation, and any difficult, unusual or complex areas highlighted.

| Services and plant areas
Many of these systems, especially on larger, more complex buildings, have significant health and safety operating issues. Handover information and training needs to be clear regarding these, including safe operation of all services and machinery. It also needs to identify procedures during emergency operation and a cascade of risk control in abnormal conditions. The actual services and electrical and mechanical plant will have their own specialist commissioning and operating manuals, but the design team will still have to provide information on plant access, escape routes and emergency systems.

Having a clear statement of intent, covering things such as hours of operation, can be helpful. At some time in the future the client may well want to operate the building for longer, but they need to be made aware that this may have safety implications, eg for security lighting. Such changes can contribute to a reduction in personal safety for the building's occupants. Consultation during this phase – such as within a 'soft landings' process (see below) – between the client and the design team may well identify these issues and generate a plan for their resolution.

## Soft Landings

Soft Landings is an approach developed by BSRIA that focuses on the most beneficial approach to handover and occupation of a new building. It also aims to ensure that as much as possible is learned from the initial handover so that future projects will benefit, effectively analysing the project to create a better briefing for the next one.

The UK Government has developed the Government Soft Landings (GSL) methodology (based on the BSRIA Soft Landings principles) for use on government projects.

The GSL methodology analyses the building under the following areas:

I Functionality and effectiveness
Meeting the needs of the occupiers and providing an effective and productive working environment.

I Environment
Meeting government performance targets in energy efficiency, water usage and waste production.

I Facilities management
A clear, cost-efficient strategy for managing the operations of the building.

I Commissioning, training and handover
Delivering and handing over the building and supporting the needs of the end users.

The GSL methodology uses good practice processes and principles that can be recommended for all projects. Both approaches are aligned with the use of BIM, both in the handover and post-occupancy phases.

### Soft Landings

BSRIA Soft Landings can be found at: bsria@bsria.co.uk

Government Soft Landings to be found at: www.bim-level2.org

## Review of Project Performance

Post-occupancy Evaluation is generally carried out during the In Use stage (see page 200: Stage 7), but it can be conducted immediately after handover (or during an extended handover period) to assess whether the initial Project Performance is as planned.

Some performance information will not be available at this stage (eg a full year's operation will be required to assess annual maintenance programmes), but based on Feedback from the building's users or the project team, the evaluation might identify some health and safety issues that can be acted upon immediately.

The Handover Strategy should include a system for dealing with such issues, based on a risk hierarchy:

I Life threatening – hopefully very rare
I Highly dangerous – there is an immediate threat that an accident will occur unless action is taken
I Dangerous – can be controlled or managed, eg by placing a cordon around the problem, allowing remedial action to be undertaken safely
I Unanticipated risk – can be approached by safeguarding the issue, then working through a remedial plan.

The strategy should include procedures for dealing with such issues and identify who will be responsible for their resolution.

## Project Information update

It can be a challenge to keep the Project Information updated at this stage, which is particularly important when computer-aided facilities management systems are adopted. However, it is important to make sure that the core information requirements are in place and updated. This will be made easier if the information has been updated regularly during the project.

The client must have a comprehensive set of information that is up to date and can be used to drive the operation of the building through its entire life. The design team and construction team can then have confidence that they have done their best to ensure that all aspects of the project are understood and can be operated efficiently and safely.

Once the project is handed over, clients and owners take over elements of the information. They can instigate changes and, as a result, the level of technical robustness can vary considerably. This may mean records start to deteriorate in accuracy, which will ultimately devalue the confidence that can be placed in them. Fortunately, many clients are coming to realise this approach is short-sighted. Increasingly, if they are in possession of accurate information at handover, they will make a real effort to ensure this continues throughout the building's life.

One of the significant advantages of a BIM approach is that if the model data is kept up to date, the model can continue to be used to plan and manage safe, efficient and proportionate maintenance.

**Tips for a successful handover**

- The handover must be organised and controlled.
- Ensure the team receiving the building are advised of health and safety first.
- Make a final check on the health and safety information prior to handover.
- Ensure any last-minute changes are identified.
- Do not be pressured into signing off safety-deficient systems.
- Make occupants aware of health aspects of the design.

## Information Exchanges

Information Exchanges required for Stage 6 are as follows:

| at stage completion: updated 'As-constructed' Information
| for UK Government projects: an output of Project Information is required.

## Chapter summary

The handover and close out of any project is a challenging stage. A lot of tasks need to be managed to ensure a completed building is ready for handover, and there are many issues that can result in health and safety problems, so having a clear, methodical approach is important.

On many projects, the majority of the handover process is undertaken by the contractor. If the design team is still involved, they need to liaise closely with the contractor. It is also helpful for the client and those occupying or using the building to be involved.

Having a full handover meeting, with representation from all the project team members (the design team, the contractor and the client), can be very successful in ensuring there is full exchange of information. This should take place on site, with a formal meeting covering all the relevant issues followed by an instructional tour of the building. A series of meetings might be required on large projects, or the client may seek a full assessment of the building in use.

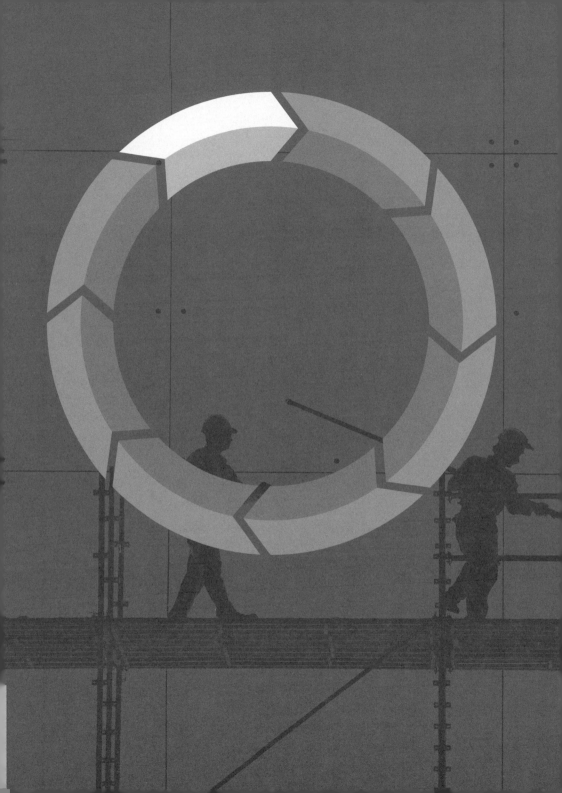

# Stage 7

# In Use

# Chapter overview

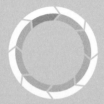

In the In Use stage of the RIBA Plan of Work 2013 it will become clear if the desired Project Outcomes set at Stage 1 have been achieved. There should be a concerted effort to understand what has been achieved: does the building or facility deliver the client's original intent and desired outcomes?

Often, however, this is not clear. Some projects change shape and direction over the course of their progress, some are subject to other influences, and some are affected by changes in the client. Whatever journey the project has been subject to, it should be understood and reviewed for the benefit of following projects.

The set-up and handover should have addressed any remaining health and safety issues. Often, however, new issues emerge as the building users become familiar with its operation. Some may arise because the building is being used differently from what was anticipated. It may also have been subject to further work, such as a fit-out operation.

Any Feedback that can be gathered following occupation can be vital in improving future projects.

**The key coverage in this chapter is as follows:**

Post-occupancy Evaluation

Updated Project Information

Follow-up

Passing on to Stage 0

Information Exchanges

# Introduction

Following handover, responsibilities for health and safety, insurance, operations, security and liabilities are in the hands of the building owner, operator and user. This is a significant change and one to be recognised, and recorded formally, by the project team. It is no longer 'their' building or their direct responsibility.

However, liability still rests with the team in certain quarters. If any risks arise, or actions occur, where the root cause is traceable back to previous design decisions, made either by the contractor or the design team, there may be liability. If the issues are of a minor nature, the client may seek compensation, but if they are of a more serious nature, resulting in actual or potential harm, the Health and Safety Executive (HSE) may seek to take action through the various measures it has at its disposal.

The HSE will investigate all serious accidents and life-critical circumstances. It will examine closely the cause of any accident, especially if there has been a fatality, and apply a tracking back procedure. This is to identify the various actions that led to the circumstances. In the case of a building this would track back how the particular elements involved in the accident were constructed and then how they were designed, picking out all of the significant decisions and who took responsibility for them during the project. This will lead to the investigators identifying the party who they think should have acted differently and could therefore have avoided the accident occurring. They may, of course, conclude that no one could have acted in a way that would have prevented the accident.

This demonstrates the need for information provided at handover for the In Use stage to be as accurate as possible, the training and commissioning to have been diligently and professionally undertaken, and the team's records of decisions made to be accurate and well organised.

*From Stage 6*

It is also important to take full advantage of the Stage 6 preparations:

A well-organised handover will normally ease the early In Use phase.

Building an understanding of how the building will be used can help.

Ensure that all health and safety functions are completely understood.

Be alert to any changes the owner or occupiers are making that may have health and safety implications.

Record for Feedback any issues that arise that could be improved by early actions.

## What are the Core Objectives of this stage?

The Core Objectives of the RIBA Plan of Work 2013 at Stage 7 are:

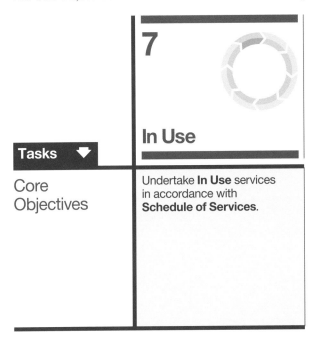

The Core Objective at this stage is to ensure that any In Use services are undertaken. These may involve completing the building handover, recording the Project Performance, making sure that all certification and testing verification and commissioning data is complete, and gathering Feedback for the benefit of future projects. Some Soft Landings activities may also be continued through this stage.

## Post-occupancy Evaluation

An area coming under increasing focus is the performance of buildings in use. In the past, the actual performance of new buildings has often not been measured. Unless there is an obvious problem, such as a leaking roof or a component failure, the performance in use is overlooked. As the measurement of all aspects of building performance has become more sophisticated, clients are demanding more – in particular, that designed performance equates to that delivered.

This applies equally to the health and safety elements of the design and construction. As health and safety supports the building in use, the health and safety record of the building after occupation is as important as its energy performance or other outcomes.

Post-occupancy Evaluation processes are set up at this point to assess Project Performance against the Project Objectives established in the initial project stages.

### Health outcomes

It will be valuable to assess health outcomes over the life of the completed building. However, this may be difficult due to confidentially issues. Many health and environment-related matters go unaddressed simply due to lack of accurate information and good quality Feedback. Internal air quality is one area of particular note.

### Indoor air quality

As buildings become more airtight, for energy conservation objectives, internal air quality can become poorer as a result. Concerns over increased levels of indoor pollutants are currently being researched. Creating sufficient levels of fresh air and avoiding materials that generate volatile organic compounds is a good starting point. When better information is available, it may well lead to more attention being given to this area.

## Safety outcomes

While health issues may be difficult to examine, the physical issues can be more straightforward. The Post-occupancy Evaluation should include reviews of the performance of the safety systems and the Feedback from the users of those systems. Some issues can only be properly understood after a full range of seasonal activities, therefore most evaluations include several visits, spaced out over several months or even a few years. However, the process must be proportional to the project and be realistic.

## The effects of changes

In the past, changes to newly completed buildings, whether due to changing requirements or tenants' needs, or simply to address shortcomings not identified in the main project, have been the cause of significant risk. These alterations are often undertaken without any real understanding of the building and without appropriate mobilisation, and many operations are extremely challenging when attempted on a finished building. Reviewing and understanding these changes can be extremely important, but achieving an understanding with the client and their team of the value in this process is often challenging. Often these issues may be seen as design shortcomings unless there is a continued relationship between the client and the design team.

### Health and safety in occupancy

- Many buildings have suffered from 'sick building syndrome'. Post-occupancy Evaluation can often help with this. Analysis of problems reported in completed buildings has revealed a number of common issues, including: too little or too dry fresh air, outgassing of chemicals from various finishes, and high-frequency flicker from some types of lighting.
- Changes to the way that the building is used can also cause problems – increased occupancy levels can put the air supply under strain, or reversed flow can make doors difficult to open.
- Everyday maintenance operations can also have safety implications – overzealous and inappropriate floor cleaning can leave a perfectly safe floor dangerously slippery.
- Many problems occur in limited areas of a building and are relatively straightforward to correct once the issue is identified.

## Updated Project Information

The Project Information is likely to require updating over the In Use phase of the building, as changes to its fabric and operation are made. If at all possible, the new information should be pulled together as a complete set of coherent information. Commonly, resources and time do not allow this process to be undertaken sufficiently thoroughly by the design team, unless as a separate commission. However, this is in everyone's interests.

### BIM methodology

Using a Building Information Modelling (BIM) methodology, it is possible at handover to provide the client with a complete and reliable model of the whole project. This can be developed by the client's team and incorporated into a computer-aided facilities management system, for use in monitoring performance and managing maintenance processes during the In Use phase.

Keeping on top of maintenance is a significant factor in ensuring 'in use' risks are kept to a minimum. The rapid growth of BIM and the development of its use in completed buildings promises to bring significant improvement in health and safety management.

### UK Government projects

On UK Government projects for this stage a formal Information Exchange is required to be undertaken.

### Computer-aided facilities management

A publicly available specification (PAS) has been published for BIM-based facilities management processes: PAS1192-3: 2014 *Specification for information management for the operational phase of assets using building information modelling.*

## Follow-up

Follow-up can usefully be continued for several years past handover and can be beneficial for both sides. As well as helping the client to resolve issues arising from how the building is being used, it may strengthen the relationship between the parties if the client feels they are being looked after.

The kind of issues that can occur are often simple, but have the potential to cause real harm. For example:

I  replacing the cleaning contractor can affect the methods used, eg a change in the type of floor polish used can create a risk of slipping
I  a change in maintenance personnel may, if they do not receive a full briefing as they take over, result in unsafe use of equipment or damage to building systems.

Simple periodic follow-up can help resolve these issues quickly and efficiently. These can also lead the client to thinking about the next project, and who would be best to be involved.

## Passing on to Stage 0

Raising standards in health and safety is largely based on making small incremental improvements, but it is also about changing a culture as well as changing actions. Pulling together information and lessons learned is a key principle of the RIBA Plan of Work 2013 – identifying what has worked on one project and, equally, what has not worked so well and needs improvement provides valuable Feedback for the next.

During Stage 7, observations that would be relevant to a new project should be collated, perhaps in a table. These can cover procedures, information, approaches, team behaviours, particular construction techniques, design details and many more issues. If recorded clearly, ideas can be reused to work towards even better performance on the next project.

## What has worked?

It is helpful to list the principal areas of the project and to set out for each what worked well (and what did not). For example:

- Client: Briefing, communication, instructions
- Brief: Clarity, delivery, realism
- Site: Picked up missing issues, capturing everything
- Team: Communication, health and safety approaches, good ideas

The key headings can be broken down into more detailed subcategories.

## Information Exchanges

Information Exchanges required for Stage 7 are as follows:

I at stage completion: updated 'As-constructed' Information, in response to ongoing client Feedback and maintenance or operational developments

I for UK Government projects: an output of Project Information may be required.

## Chapter summary     7

The use of Stage 7 as a driver to achieving a full understanding of the building in use is a significant advance in several areas. The benefits for health and safety in particular are considerable. Ensuring that the building is managed and operated as designed and that all equipment is used as intended will enable the health and safety objectives to be fully realised.

In the past, the lack of involvement of the design team in the In Use phase has resulted in risks being generated or building occupants being exposed to unnecessary risk. The full application of this stage could see this come to an end.

# Appendix 1: The Construction (Design and Management) Regulations 2015

In 2007, the new version of the CDM regulations changed several principles that were thought to be troublesome in the version previously in place. In particular, they replaced the planning supervisor role with the CDM coordinator (the CDM-C), they changed some definitions and, as the HSE said at the time, they made explicit areas that had previously been implied.

There was a commitment to review the regulations in three years. By that time it was clear to many that the new regulations were not quite as successful as had been hoped.

Several difficult points had opened up. In particular, there was growing pressure from the EU as the UK had not fully implemented EU Council Directive 92/57/EEC (on temporary or mobile construction sites), the role of the CDM-C was still not achieving what had been hoped, and the industry was drowning in paperwork as a result of misinterpretation, preventing the regulations from being as effective as intended. A consultation confirmed that, while the actual regulations were thought by everyone – government, regulators and industry – to be right in principle, implementation was reducing their effectiveness.

Following the consultation, a number of initiatives – such as the Löfstedt review and the Red Tape Challenge – delayed the development of revised regulations until 2014. Following further revisions the regulations were issued in early 2015, hopefully heralding a new and more effective approach. In parallel, many in the industry are also hoping that a new realism can accompany the regulations. In support of this the HSE is working closely with industry to help ensure that unintended consequences are kept to a minimum.

## The 2015 CDM regulations

The 2015 regulations addressed a number of issues:

I   full implementation of the EU directive, in particular with the introduction of the domestic client and revised thresholds of notification
I   removal of the CDM-C role
I   addition of the principal designer role (to balance the principal contractor role)
I   reduction in bureaucracy, principally by changing the direct competency requirements
I   more focus on small sites, especially in respect of falls, refurbishment and plant accidents
I   measures to ensure the protection for workers is not diminished
I   simplification of the regulations' structure, to follow the natural process of a project.

**Statutory Instrument: 2015 No. 51**

The Construction (Design and Management) Regulations 2015

Laid before Parliament    29 January 2015

Came into force        6 April 2015

The CDM regulations are structured as follows:

PART 1 Introduction
Regulation 1    Citation and commencement
Regulation 2    Interpretation
Regulation 3    Application in and outside Great Britain

PART 2 Client duties
Regulation 4    Client duties in relation to managing projects
Regulation 5    Appointment of the principal designer and the principal contractor
Regulation 6    Notification
Regulation 7    Application to domestic clients

Schedule 1    Particulars to be notified under regulation 6
Schedule 2    Minimum welfare facilities required for construction sites
Schedule 3    Work involving particular risks
Schedule 4    Transitional and saving provisions
Schedule 5    Amendments

## Key changes commentary 2007–2015

Directly reflecting the scope of the EU directive has been a challenge for the HSE, although it remains to be seen if the European Commission agrees that the 2015 changes achieve full implementation. The Commission has embarked on a review of the effectiveness of current health and safety legislation, although the timetable may mean any implications are not seen for several years.

Additionally, the 2015 changes set out to simplify the regulations and remove any 'goldplating', discouraging bureaucracy and promoting the use of better regulatory principles.

The removal of the CDM-C role and the addition of the principal designer role is significant. The concept behind this is that this new position balances that of the principal contractor: one in authority over the pre-construction phase, one in authority over the construction phase. The principal designer is in a more strategic role, acting from 'inside' the design team. The main concern is to ensure that the pre-construction phase activities are addressing the right issues and producing the right information; the role is less about developing detailed procedures and more about being an integrated and influencing force, with an ability to understand design nuances.

The changes to the thresholds for notification mean there is now one simple formula. Notification is required for projects scheduled to last more than 30 working days and have more than 20 workers working at any one time, or which will exceed 500 person days.

Domestic clients are now included within the regulations, under the provisions to fully implement the EU directive. The domestic client position has been carefully formulated:

| If there is only one contractor, the client duties and the contractor duties are undertaken by the contractor.
| If a domestic client employs more than one contractor then the contractor duties and the client duties fall on the contractor that has been appointed as the principal contractor. It the client fails to appoint a principal contractor, the duties fall on the contractor in charge of the project.
| A domestic client also has the option, to be agreed in writing, that a designer can be asked to undertake the client duties. This is often the approach that naturally fits a small domestic project.

## Competence

The focus on regulating competence has given rise to an industry providing checking services, which has become disproportionate to the original intentions. (These details were covered in Appendix 4 of the 2007 regulations, which has been withdrawn from the 2015 version.) The HSE is looking to professional institutions and other organisations to provide the guidance and administration needed to ensure competence. The HSE is keen to liaise with industry as to how this will develop.

The HSE feels that a fully qualified chartered architect or architectural technologist with a wide range of experience (at least three years) and with up-to-date CPD should have the necessary skills, knowledge and experience to undertake the principal designer role. Their experience should be across a range of projects and contracts, and for some of that time they should have been leading a project. It should also include working with colleagues who are considerably more experienced.

# Appendix 2: The workplace regulations incorporated as part of the 2015 CDM regulations

Following the revision to the CDM regulations in 2007, the Workplace (Health, Safety and Welfare) Regulations 1992 (SI 1992 No. 3004, the 'workplace regulations') were incorporated into those regulations. They are a set of basic provisions that are largely covered either by Building Regulations or under the remit of building owners and operators.

The workplace regulations continue to cause problems, however, as many clients and procurement assessment bodies take the view that design consultants should know them and ensure they are covered in projects and designs. The problem is that not all the provisions are covered elsewhere and therefore designers need to have an understanding of the regulations.

Equally, though, non-designers need to be clear that the provisions of these regulations are met by other means, either by compliance with Building Regulations, through professional competence or simply by providing a service to an acceptable level.

## The workplace regulations: scope

Consultants need to be aware of the implications of the workplace regulations and respond accordingly, if appropriate.

The workplace regulations are structured as follows:

Regulation 1     Citation and commencement
Regulation 2     Interpretation
Regulation 3     Application
Regulation 4     Requirements
Regulation 5     Maintenance of workplace, and of equipment, devices and systems
Regulation 6     Ventilation
Regulation 7     Temperature in indoor workplaces

| | |
|---|---|
| Regulation 8 | Lighting |
| Regulation 9 | Cleanliness and waste materials |
| Regulation 10 | Room dimensions and space |
| Regulation 11 | Workstations and seating |
| Regulation 12 | Condition of floors and traffic routes |
| Regulation 13 | Falls or falling objects |
| Regulation 14 | Windows, and transparent or translucent doors, gates and walls |
| Regulation 15 | Windows, skylights and ventilators |
| Regulation 16 | Ability to clean windows etc safely |
| Regulation 17 | Organisation etc of traffic routes |
| Regulation 18 | Doors and gates |
| Regulation 19 | Escalators and moving walkways |
| Regulation 20 | Sanitary conveniences |
| Regulation 21 | Washing facilities |
| Regulation 22 | Drinking water |
| Regulation 23 | Accommodation for clothing |
| Regulation 24 | Facilities for changing clothing |
| Regulation 25 | Facilities to rest and eat meals |
| Regulation 26 | Exemption certificates |
| Regulation 27 | Repeals, saving and revocations |
| Schedule 1 | Provisions applicable to factories which are not new workplaces, extensions or conversions |
| Schedule 2 | Repeals and revocations |

## Guidance notes

The relevant regulatory requirements are laid out below.

### Regulation 5    Maintenance of workplace, and of equipment, devices and systems

(1) The workplace and the equipment, devices and systems to which this regulation applies shall be maintained (including cleaned as appropriate) in an efficient state, in efficient working order and in good repair.

(2) Where appropriate, the equipment, devices and systems to which this regulation applies shall be subject to a suitable system of maintenance.

(3) The equipment, devices and systems to which this regulation applies are –

(a) equipment and devices a fault in which is liable to result in a failure to comply with any of these Regulations; and

(b) mechanical ventilation systems provided pursuant to regulation 6 (whether or not they include equipment or devices within sub-paragraph (a) of this paragraph).

*Commentary*
This is an issue for the operators and owners of buildings. Under the CDM regulations, the design must be capable of safe maintenance.

Rarely within a design consultant's scope, but may be within the scope of interior designers and mechanical and electrical engineers.

**Regulation 6    Ventilation**
(1) Effective and suitable provision shall be made to ensure that every enclosed workplace is ventilated by a sufficient quantity of fresh or purified air.

(2) Any plant used for the purpose of complying with paragraph (1) shall include an effective device to give visible or audible warning of any failure of the plant where necessary for reasons of health or safety.

(3) This Regulation shall not apply to any enclosed workplace or part of a workplace which is subject to the provisions of –
 (a) section 30 of the Factories Act 1961;
 (b) regulations 49 to 52 of the Shipbuilding and Ship-Repairing Regulations 1960;
 (c) regulation 21 of the Construction (General Provisions) Regulations 1961;
 (d) regulation 18 of the Docks Regulations 1988.

*Commentary*
Natural ventilation and simple mechanical ventilation requirements are covered by Building Regulations approved document (AD) F.

Mechanical ventilation of a complex nature must be designed by a mechanical engineer.

**Regulation 7    Temperature in indoor workplaces**
(1) During working hours, the temperature in all workplaces inside buildings shall be reasonable.

(2) A method of heating or cooling shall not be used which results in the escape into a workplace of fumes, gas or vapour of such

character and to such extent that they are likely to be injurious or offensive to any person.

(3) A sufficient number of thermometers shall be provided to enable persons at work to determine the temperature in any workplace inside a building.

*Commentary*
This is covered by Building Regulations ADs J and L.

Whether the actual temperature is delivered will rely on the building operator or owner ensuring that the systems are set correctly. There may occasionally be a performance issue with new buildings. This is why we advocate use of the 'soft landings' principles.

**Regulation 8    Lighting**
(1) Every workplace shall have suitable and sufficient lighting.
(2) The lighting mentioned in paragraph (1) shall, so far as is reasonably practicable, be by natural light.
(3) Without prejudice to the generality of paragraph (1), suitable and sufficient emergency lighting shall be provided in any room in circumstances in which persons at work are specially exposed to danger in the event of failure of artificial lighting.

*Commentary*
Natural lighting is covered by planning and Building Regulations requirements (AD M)

Design performance of artificial lighting is covered by an electrical engineer, with some input from the architect and the interior designer, mainly to supply data explaining the design.

This is not a subject that a designer could ever ignore or omit.

**Regulation 9    Cleanliness and waste materials**
(1) Every workplace and the furniture, furnishings and fittings therein shall be kept sufficiently clean.
(2) The surfaces of the floors, walls and ceilings of all workplaces inside buildings shall be capable of being kept sufficiently clean.
(3) So far as is reasonably practicable, waste materials shall not be allowed to accumulate in a workplace except in suitable receptacles.

*Commentary*
Designing for safe cleaning and waste disposal is required by the CDM regulations. Ensuring this happens, however, is within the remit of the building owner and operator.

Workplaces are required to have provision for waste under Building Regulations Regulation 7 and AD H.

## Regulation 10   Room dimensions and space

(1) Every room where persons work shall have sufficient floor area, height and unoccupied space for purposes of health, safety and welfare.
(2) It shall be sufficient compliance with this regulation in a workplace which is not a new workplace, a modification, an extension or a conversion and which, immediately before this regulation came into force in respect of it, was subject to the provisions of the Factories Act 1961, if the workplace does not contravene the provisions of Part I of Schedule 1.

*Commentary*
All spaces have to be designed with care and professional competence and apply a common sense approach.

This is not a subject that any designer should ever ignore.

## Regulation 11   Workstations and seating

(1) Every workstation shall be so arranged that it is suitable both for any person at work in the workplace who is likely to work at that workstation and for any work of the undertaking which is likely to be done there.
(2) Without prejudice to the generality of paragraph (1), every workstation outdoors shall be so arranged that –
    (a) so far as is reasonably practicable, it provides protection from adverse weather;
    (b) it enables any person at the workstation to leave it swiftly or, as appropriate, to be assisted in the event of an emergency; and
    (c) it ensures that any person at the workstation is not likely to slip or fall.
(3) A suitable seat shall be provided for each person at work in the workplace whose work includes operations of a kind that the work (or a substantial part of it) can or must be done sitting.

(4) A seat shall not be suitable for the purposes of paragraph (3) unless –

   (a) it is suitable for the person for whom it is provided as well as for the operations to be performed; and

   (b) a suitable footrest is also provided where necessary.

*Commentary*

Often this will not form part of an architectural design commission. Where it does apply, it will be part of an interior design commission and fundamental to the designer.

**Regulation 12   Condition of floors and traffic routes**

(1) Every floor in a workplace and the surface of every traffic route in a workplace shall be of a construction such that the floor or surface of the traffic route is suitable for the purpose for which it is used.

(2) Without prejudice to the generality of paragraph (1), the requirements in that paragraph shall include requirements that –

   (a) the floor, or surface of the traffic route, shall have no hole or slope, or be uneven or slippery so as, in each case, to expose any person to a risk to his health or safety; and

   (b) every such floor shall have effective means of drainage where necessary.

(3) So far as is reasonably practicable, every floor in a workplace and the surface of every traffic route in a workplace shall be kept free from obstructions and from any article or substance which may cause a person to slip, trip or fall.

(4) In considering whether for the purposes of paragraph (2) (a) a hole or slope exposes any person to a risk to his health or safety –

   (a) no account shall be taken of a hole where adequate measures have been taken to prevent a person falling; and

   (b) account shall be taken of any handrail provided in connection with any slope,

(5) Suitable and sufficient handrails and, if appropriate, guards shall be provided on all traffic routes which are staircases except in circumstances in which a handrail can not be provided without obstructing the traffic route.

*Commentary*

Partly covered by Building Regulations Regulation 7 and ADs K and M.

Appropriate use of materials and slips and trips form part of core design considerations.

### Regulation 13   Falls or falling objects

(1)   So far as is reasonably practicable, suitable and effective measures shall be taken to prevent any event specified in paragraph (3).

(2)   So far as is reasonably practicable, the measures required by paragraph (1) shall be measures other than the provision of personal protective equipment, information, instruction, training or supervision.

(3)   The events specified in this paragraph are –
    (a)   any person falling a distance likely to cause personal injury;
    (b)   any person being struck by a falling object likely to cause personal injury.

(4)   Any area where there is a risk to health or safety from any event mentioned in paragraph (3) shall be clearly indicated where appropriate.

(5)   So far as is practicable, every tank, pit or structure where there is a risk of a person in the workplace falling into a dangerous substance in the tank, pit or structure, shall be securely covered or fenced.

(6)   Every traffic route over, across or in an uncovered tank, pit or structure such as is mentioned in paragraph (5) shall be securely fenced.

(7)   In this Regulation, 'dangerous substance' means –
    (a)   any substance likely to scald or burn;
    (b)   any poisonous substance;
    (c)   any corrosive substance;
    (d)   any fume, gas or vapour likely to overcome a person; or
    (e)   any granular or free flowing solid substance, or any viscous substance which, in any case, is of a nature or quantity which is likely to cause danger to any person.

*Commentary*
Partly covered by Building Regulations AD K.

Industrial and manufacturing elements covered by structural, process and chemical engineers.

### Regulation 14    Windows, and transparent or translucent doors, gates and walls

(1)  Every window or other transparent or translucent surface in a wall or partition and every transparent or translucent surface in a door or gate shall, where necessary for reasons of health or safety –

(a)  be of safety material or be protected against breakage of the transparent or translucent material; and

(b)  be appropriately marked or incorporate features so as, in either case, to make it apparent.

*Commentary*
Covered by Building Regulations Regulation 7 and AD K.

### Regulation 15    Windows, skylights and ventilators

(1)  No window, skylight or ventilator which is capable of being opened shall be likely to be opened, closed or adjusted in a manner which exposes any person performing such operation to a risk to his health or safety.

(2)  No window, skylight or ventilator shall be in a position when open which is likely to expose any person in the workplace to a risk to his health or safety.

*Commentary*
Covered by Building Regulations Regulation 7 and AD K.

### Regulation 16    Ability to clean windows etc safely

(1)  All windows and skylights in a workplace shall be of a design or be so constructed that they may be cleaned safely.

(2)  In considering whether a window or skylight is of a design or so constructed as to comply with paragraph (1), account may be taken of equipment used in conjunction with the window or skylight or of devices fitted to the building.

*Commentary*
Covered by Building Regulations Regulation 7 and AD K.

### Regulation 17    Organisation etc of traffic routes

(1)  Every workplace shall be organised in such a way that pedestrians and vehicles can circulate in a safe manner.

(2)  Traffic routes in a workplace shall be suitable for the persons or vehicles using them, sufficient in number, in suitable positions and of sufficient size.

(3)  Without prejudice to the generality of paragraph (2), traffic routes shall not satisfy the requirements of that paragraph unless suitable measures are taken to ensure that –
   (a)  pedestrians or, as the case may be, vehicles may use a traffic route without causing danger to the health or safety of persons at work near it;
   (b)  there is sufficient separation of any traffic route for vehicles from doors or gates or from traffic routes for pedestrians which lead onto it; and
   (c)  where vehicles and pedestrians use the same traffic route, there is sufficient separation between them.
(4)  All traffic routes shall be suitably indicated where necessary for reasons of health or safety.
(5)  Paragraph (2) shall apply so far as is reasonably practicable, to a workplace which is not a new workplace, a modification, an extension or a conversion.

*Commentary*
Not something to be ignored, but also not something design consultants would have control over. Planning authorities and highways and civil engineers will have more involvement.

### Regulation 18   Doors and gates
(1)  Doors and gates shall be suitably constructed (including being fitted with any necessary safety devices).
(2)  Without prejudice to the generality of paragraph (1), doors and gates shall not comply with that paragraph unless –
   (a)  any sliding door or gate has a device to prevent it coming off its track during use;
   (b)  any upward opening door or gate has a device to prevent it falling back;
   (c)  any powered door or gate has suitable and effective features to prevent it causing injury by trapping any person;
   (d)  where necessary for reasons of health or safety, any powered door or gate can be operated manually unless it opens automatically if the power fails; and
   (e)  any door or gate which is capable of opening by being pushed from either side is of such a construction as to provide, when closed, a clear view of the space close to both sides.

*Commentary*
Part of normal design considerations as necessary and practical. Part of fitness for purpose under Building Regulations Regulation 7.

### Regulation 19   Escalators and moving walkways
(1)  Escalators and moving walkways shall –
   (a)   function safely;
   (b)   be equipped with any necessary safety devices;
   (c)   be fitted with one or more emergency stop controls which are easily identifiable and readily accessible.

*Commentary*
Not part of an architect's remit, but may be part of a service engineer's remit.

### Regulation 20   Sanitary conveniences
(1)  Suitable and sufficient sanitary conveniences shall be provided at readily accessible places.
(2)  Without prejudice to the generality of paragraph (1), sanitary conveniences shall not be suitable unless –
   (a)   the rooms containing them are adequately ventilated and lit;
   (b)   they and the rooms containing them are kept in a clean and orderly condition; and
   (c)   separate rooms containing conveniences are provided for men and women except where and so far as each convenience is in a separate room the door of which is capable of being secured from inside.
(3)  It shall be sufficient compliance with the requirements in paragraph (1) to provide sufficient sanitary conveniences in a workplace which is not a new workplace, a modification, an extension or a conversion and which, immediately before this regulation came into force in respect of it, was subject to the provisions of the Factories Act 1961, if sanitary conveniences are provided in accordance with the provisions of Part II of Schedule 1.

*Commentary*
Covered by Building Regulations Regulation 7 and ADs H and M.

### Regulation 21    Washing facilities

(1)  Suitable and sufficient washing facilities, including showers if required by the nature of the work or for health reasons, shall be provided at readily accessible places.

(2)  Without prejudice to the generality of paragraph (1), washing facilities shall not be suitable unless –
- (a)  they are provided in the immediate vicinity of every sanitary convenience, whether or not provided elsewhere as well;
- (b)  they are provided in the vicinity of any changing rooms required by these regulations, whether or not provided elsewhere as well;
- (c)  they include a supply of clean hot and cold, or warm, water (which shall be running water so far as is practicable);
- (d)  they include soap or other suitable means of cleaning;
- (e)  they include towels or other suitable means of drying;
- (f)  the rooms containing them are sufficiently ventilated and lit;
- (g)  they and the rooms containing them are kept in a clean and orderly condition; and
- (h)  separate facilities are provided for men and women, except where and so far as they are provided in a room the door of which is capable of being secured from inside and the facilities in each such room are intended to be used by only one person at a time.

(3)  Paragraph (2)(h) shall not apply to facilities which are provided for washing hands, forearms and face only.

*Commentary*
Covered by Building Regulations ADs F, H and G.

### Regulation 22    Drinking water

(1)  An adequate supply of wholesome drinking water shall be provided for all persons at work in the workplace.

(2)  Every supply of drinking water required by paragraph (1) shall –
- (a)  be readily accessible at suitable places; and
- (b)  be conspicuously marked by an appropriate sign where necessary for reasons of health and safety.

(3)  Where a supply of drinking water is required by paragraph (1), there shall also be provided a sufficient number of suitable cups or other drinking vessels unless the supply of drinking water is in a jet from which persons can drink easily.

*Commentary*
Part of a mechanical engineer's remit.

### Regulation 23   Accommodation for clothing

(1)  Suitable and sufficient accommodation shall be provided –

    (a)  for the clothing of any person at work which is not worn during working hours; and

    (b)  for special clothing which is worn by any person at work but which is not taken home.

(2)  Without prejudice to the generality of paragraph (1), the accommodation mentioned in that paragraph shall not be suitable unless –

    (a)  where facilities to change clothing are required by regulation 24, it provides suitable security for the clothing mentioned in paragraph (1) (a);

    (b)  where necessary to avoid risks to health or damage to the clothing, it includes separate accommodation for clothing worn at work and for other clothing;

    (c)  so far as is reasonably practicable, it allows or includes facilities for drying clothing; and

    (d)  it is in a suitable location.

*Commentary*
Not part of a design consultant's remit.

### Regulation 24   Facilities for changing clothing

(1)  Suitable and sufficient facilities shall be provided for any person at work in the workplace to change clothing in all cases where –

    (a)  the person has to wear special clothing for the purpose of work; and

    (b)  the person can not, for reasons of health or propriety, be expected to change in another room.

(2)  Without prejudice to the generality of paragraph (1), the facilities mentioned in that paragraph shall not be suitable unless they include separate facilities for, or separate use of facilities by, men and women where necessary for reasons of propriety.

*Commentary*
Not often part of a design consultant's remit.

**Regulation 25   Facilities for rest and to eat meals**
(1)   Suitable and sufficient rest facilities shall be provided at readily accessible places.
(2)   Rest facilities provided by virtue of paragraph (1) shall –
   (a)   where necessary for reasons of health or safety include, in the case of a new workplace, an extension or a conversion, rest facilities provided in one or more rest rooms, or, in other cases, in rest rooms or rest areas;
   (b)   include suitable facilities to eat meals where food eaten in the workplace would otherwise be likely to become contaminated.
(3)   Rest rooms and rest areas shall include suitable arrangements to protect non-smokers from discomfort caused by tobacco smoke.
(4)   Suitable facilities shall be provided for any person at work who is a pregnant woman or nursing mother to rest.
(5)   Suitable and sufficient facilities shall be provided for persons at work to eat meals where meals are regularly eaten in the workplace.

*Commentary*
Part of the normal design considerations when within the brief.

## References

*Workplace health, safety and welfare. Workplace (Health, Safety and Welfare) Regulations 1992. Approved Code of Practice and guidance (L24)*
Health and Safety Executive, 2013 (2nd edition), HSE Books, ISBN: 9780717665839.

# Appendix 3: Risk evaluation templates

The following are suggested for use in recording and tracking project risks. However, they may need to be modified to suit the project and contractual arrangements.

|   The forms are used during design development and circulated between consultants to ensure that key risks are identified, discussed and resolved. This may be by revising the design or by adopting controls and special measures.
|   The progress is summarised in the summary template.
|   The concluding information is issued to the construction team.
|   The drawn information is probably the most important and should be clear, accurate and concise.

## Risk design evaluation process summary template

| Project: | | | Project no.: | | Work stage: | Date: | Rev: |
|---|---|---|---|---|---|---|---|
| Risk ref / Date opened | Element or activity and hazard or potential to cause harm | Persons at risk, likelihood of risk | Design team Risk Reduction Proposals required to mitigate the risk (with options/ alternatives recorded) | Responsibilities and actions | | | |
| | | | | Required date of action or work stage | Risk closed, open or residual | Risk action owner | |
| Example 1 | | | | | | | |
| Example 2 | | | | | | | |
| Example 3 etc | | | | | | | |

## Risk design evaluation process template

| Project: | | | Project no.: | | Work stage: | Date: | Rev: |
|---|---|---|---|---|---|---|---|
| Risk ref / Date opened | Element or activity and hazard or potential to cause harm | Persons at risk, likelihood of risk | Design team Risk Reduction Proposals required to mitigate the risk (with options/ alternatives recorded) | Responsibilities and actions | | | |
| | | | | Required date of action or work stage | Risk closed, open or residual | Risk action owner | |
| Details | | | | | | | |
| Location drawing or general arrangement | | | | | Detailed drawing | | |

# Further reading

## HSE publications

HSG 65: *Managing for health and safety*, 2013 (3rd edn)

HSG 150: *Health and safety in construction*, 2006

HSG 168: *Fire safety in construction*, 2010

HSG 263: *Involving your workforce in health and safety: Good practice for all workplaces*, 2008

L24: *Workplace health, safety and welfare. Workplace (Health, Safety and Welfare) Regulations 1992. Approved Code of Practice and guidance*, 2013 (2nd edn)

## Books

*Safety Can't Be Measured: An Evidence-based Approach to Improving Risk Reduction*
Andrew Townsend, 2013, Gower

*A Practical Guide to Public Procurement*
Abby Semple, 2015, Oxford University Press

*CDM 2015: A Practical Guide for Architects and Designers*
Paul Bussey, 2015, RIBA Publishing

## Standards and specifications

| | |
|---|---|
| BS 1192-4: 2014 | *Collaborative production of information. Fulfilling employer's information exchange requirements using COBie. Code of practice* |
| PAS 91:2013 | *Construction prequalification questionnaires* |
| BS EN ISO 9001: 2015 | *Quality management systems. Requirements* |

BS EN ISO 9004: 2009    *Managing for the sustained success of an organization. A quality management approach*

PAS 1192-2: 2013    *Specification for information management for the capital/delivery phase of construction projects using building information modelling*

PAS 1192-3: 2014    *Specification for information management for the operational phase of assets using building information modelling*

# Health and safety glossary

### Approved code of practice (ACOP)

Officially produced guidance on the implementation of statutory requirements. ACOPs are not legally enforceable, but are given weight by the courts in any proceedings.

### Buildability

A term used to describe a construction design or detail that can be undertaken in a safe and practical manner.

### CDM regulations

The Construction (Design and Management) Regulations 2015 (or earlier edition if specifically stated).

### Domestic client

A client for whom a project is not being carried out in the course of their business, as defined in the CDM regulations. Additional duties apply on projects with a domestic client

### EU directive

Council Directive 92/57/EEC on the implementation of minimum safety and health requirements at temporary or mobile construction sites.

### Fire safety order

Regulatory Reform (Fire Safety) Order 2005.

### Health and Safety Executive (HSE)

Statutory authority with responsibility for enforcing health and safety legislation in the UK.

### Health and safety file

Required under the CDM regulations.

### HSWA

The Health and Safety at Work etc Act 1974.

### IRATA

The Industrial Rope Access Trade Association.

### PPE

Personal protective equipment.

### Pre-construction information

Required under the CDM regulations.

### Principal contractor

Role required under the CDM regulations, referring to the contractor who has responsibility for the works.

### Principal designer

Role required under the CDM regulations. referring to the designer who has authority over the design and for the purposes of the CDM regulations has responsibilities for management of safe design.

### Procurement

The collective term referring to the selection process involved in a project. This concerns the selection of the team, the contractor's supply chain and materials.

### Schedule 3 (to the CDM regulations)

A list of types of work involving particular risks, for which specific health and safety measures are required.

### 'so far as is reasonably practicable' (SFARP)

A level of obligation placed on dutyholders in particular (such as the principal designer, client and principal contractor). It requires the level of risk and measures applied to control risk in terms of money, time and resources to be balanced.

It covers all duties covered by the CDM regulations. It is not an absolute criterion.

**Soft Landings**

A methodology for optimising the handover and post-occupation activities, to improve

the use of the building and lead to improvements on future projects.

**SSIP**

Safety Schemes in Procurement: the organisation that coordinates construction industry prequalification schemes.

**Workplace regulations**

The Workplace (Health, Safety and Welfare) Regulations 1992.

# RIBA Plan of Work 2013 glossary

A number of new themes and subject matters have been included in the RIBA Plan of Work 2013. The following presents a glossary of all of the capitalised terms that are used throughout the RIBA Plan of Work 2013. Defining certain terms has been necessary to clarify the intent of a term, to provide additional insight into the purpose of certain terms and to ensure consistency in the interpretation of the RIBA Plan of Work 2013.

### 'As-constructed' Information

Information produced at the end of a project to represent what has been constructed. This will comprise a mixture of 'as-built' information from specialist subcontractors and the 'final construction issue' from design team members. Clients may also wish to undertake 'as-built' surveys using new surveying technologies to bring a further degree of accuracy to this information.

### Building Contract

The contract between the client and the contractor for the construction of the project. In some instances, the **Building Contract** may contain design duties for specialist subcontractors and/or design team members. On some projects, more than one Building Contract may be required; for example, one for shell and core works and another for furniture, fitting and equipment aspects.

### Building Information Modelling (BIM)

BIM is widely used as the acronym for 'Building Information Modelling', which is commonly defined (using the Construction Project Information Committee (CPIC) definition) as: 'digital representation of physical and functional characteristics of a facility creating a shared knowledge resource for information about it and forming a reliable basis for decisions during its life cycle, from earliest conception to demolition'.

### Business Case

The **Business Case** for a project is the rationale behind the initiation of a new building project. It may consist solely of a reasoned argument. It may contain supporting information, financial appraisals or other background information. It should also highlight initial considerations for the **Project Outcomes**. In summary, it is a combination of objective and subjective considerations. The **Business Case** might be prepared in relation to, for example, appraising a number of sites or in relation to assessing a refurbishment against a new build option.

### Change Control Procedures

Procedures for controlling changes to the design and construction following the sign-off of the Stage 2 Concept Design and the **Final Project Brief**.

### Common Standards

Publicly available standards frequently used to define project and design management processes in relation to the briefing, designing, constructing, maintaining, operating and use of a building.

### Communication Strategy

The strategy that sets out when the project team will meet, how they will communicate effectively and the protocols for issuing information between the various parties, both informally and at Information Exchanges.

## Construction Programme

The period in the **Project Programme** and the **Building Contract** for the construction of the project, commencing on the site mobilisation date and ending at **Practical Completion**.

## Construction Strategy

A strategy that considers specific aspects of the design that may affect the buildability or logistics of constructing a project, or may affect health and safety aspects. The **Construction Strategy** comprises items such as cranage, site access and accommodation locations, reviews of the supply chain and sources of materials, and specific buildability items, such as the choice of frame (steel or concrete) or the installation of larger items of plant. On a smaller project, the strategy may be restricted to the location of site cabins and storage, and the ability to transport materials up an existing staircase.

## Contractor's Proposals

Proposals presented by a contractor to the client in response to a tender that includes the **Employer's Requirements**. The **Contractor's Proposals** may match the **Employer's Requirements**, although certain aspects may be varied based on value engineered solutions and additional information may be submitted to clarify what is included in the tender. The **Contractor's Proposals** form an integral component of the **Building Contract** documentation.

## Contractual Tree

A diagram that clarifies the contractual relationship between the client and the parties undertaking the roles required on a project.

## Cost Information

All of the project costs, including the cost estimate and life cycle costs where required.

## Design Programme

A programme setting out the strategic dates in relation to the design process. It is aligned with the **Project Programme** but is strategic in its nature, due to the iterative nature of the design process, particularly in the early stages.

## Design Queries

Queries relating to the design arising from the site, typically managed using a contractor's in-house request for information (RFI) or technical query (TQ) process.

## Design Responsibility Matrix

A matrix that sets out who is responsible for designing each aspect of the project and when. This document sets out the extent of any performance specified design. The **Design Responsibility Matrix** is created at a strategic level at Stage 1 and fine tuned in response to the Concept Design at the end of Stage 2 in order to ensure that there are no design responsibility ambiguities at Stages 3, 4 and 5.

## Employer's Requirements

Proposals prepared by design team members. The level of detail will depend on the stage at which the tender is issued to the contractor. The **Employer's Requirements** may comprise a mixture of prescriptive elements and descriptive elements to allow the contractor a degree of flexibility in determining the **Contractor's Proposals**.

### Feasibility Studies

Studies undertaken on a given site to test the feasibility of the **Initial Project Brief** on a specific site or in a specific context and to consider how site-wide issues will be addressed.

### Feedback

**Feedback** from the project team, including the end users, following completion of a building.

### Final Project Brief

The **Initial Project Brief** amended so that it is aligned with the Concept Design and any briefing decisions made during Stage 2. (Both the Concept Design and **Initial Project Brief** are Information Exchanges at the end of Stage 2.)

### Handover Strategy

The strategy for handing over a building, including the requirements for phased handovers, commissioning, training of staff or other factors crucial to the successful occupation of a building. On some projects, the Building Services Research and Information Association (BSRIA) Soft Landings process is used as the basis for formulating the strategy and undertaking a **Post-occupancy Evaluation** (www.bsria. co.uk/services/design/soft-landings/).

### Health and Safety Strategy

The strategy covering all aspects of health and safety on the project, outlining legislative requirements as well as other project initiatives, including the **Maintenance and Operational Strategy**.

### Information Exchange

The formal issue of information for review

and sign-off by the client at key stages of the project. The project team may also have additional formal **Information Exchanges** as well as the many informal exchanges that occur during the iterative design process.

### Initial Project Brief

The brief prepared following discussions with the client to ascertain the **Project Objectives**, the client's **Business Case** and, in certain instances, in response to site **Feasibility Studies**.

### Maintenance and Operational Strategy

The strategy for the maintenance and operation of a building, including details of any specific plant required to replace components.

### Post-occupancy Evaluation

Evaluation undertaken post occupancy to determine whether the **Project Outcomes**, both subjective and objective, set out in the **Final Project Brief** have been achieved.

### Practical Completion

**Practical Completion** is a contractual term used in the **Building Contract** to signify the date on which a project is handed over to the client. The date triggers a number of contractual mechanisms.

### Project Budget

The client's budget for the project, which may include the construction cost as well as the cost of certain items required post completion and during the project's operational use.

### Project Execution Plan

The **Project Execution Plan** is produced in collaboration between the project lead and lead designer, with contributions from other designers and members of the project team. The **Project Execution Plan** sets out the processes and protocols to be used to develop the design. It is sometimes referred to as a project quality plan.

## Project Information

Information, including models, documents, specifications, schedules and spreadsheets, issued between parties during each stage and in formal Information Exchanges at the end of each stage.

## Project Objectives

The client's key objectives as set out in the **Initial Project Brief**. The document includes, where appropriate, the employer's **Business Case**, **Sustainability Aspirations** or other aspects that may influence the preparation of the brief and, in turn, the Concept Design stage. For example, **Feasibility Studies** may be required in order to test the **Initial Project Brief** against a given site, allowing certain high-level briefing issues to be considered before design work commences in earnest.

## Project Outcomes

The desired outcomes for the project (for example, in the case of a hospital this might be a reduction in recovery times). The outcomes may include operational aspects and a mixture of subjective and objective criteria.

## Project Performance

The performance of the project, determined using **Feedback**, including about the performance of the project team and the performance of the building against the desired **Project Outcomes**.

## Project Programme

The overall period for the briefing, design, construction and post-completion activities of a project.

## Project Roles Table

A table that sets out the roles required on a project as well as defining the stages during which those roles are required and the parties responsible for carrying out the roles.

## Project Strategies

The strategies developed in parallel with the Concept Design to support the design and, in certain instances, to respond to the **Final Project Brief** as it is concluded. These strategies typically include:

I   acoustic strategy
I   fire engineering strategy
I   **Maintenance and Operational Strategy**
I   **Sustainability Strategy**
I   building control strategy
I   **Technology Strategy**.

These strategies are usually prepared in outline at Stage 2 and in detail at Stage 3, with the recommendations absorbed into the Stage 4 outputs and Information Exchanges.

The strategies are not typically used for construction purposes because they may contain recommendations or information that contradict the drawn information. The intention is that they should be transferred into the various models or drawn information.

## Quality Objectives

The objectives that set out the quality aspects of a project. The objectives may comprise both subjective and objective aspects, although subjective aspects may be subject to a design quality indicator (DQI) benchmark review during the **Feedback** period.

## Research and Development

Project-specific research and development responding to the **Initial Project Brief** or in response to the Concept Design as it is developed.

### Risk Assessment

The **Risk Assessment** considers the various design and other risks on a project and how each risk will be managed and the party responsible for managing each risk.

### Schedule of Services

A list of specific services and tasks to be undertaken by a party involved in the project which is incorporated into their professional services contract.

### Site Information

Specific **Project Information** in the form of specialist surveys or reports relating to the project- or site-specific context.

### Strategic Brief

The brief prepared to enable the Strategic Definition of the project. Strategic considerations might include considering different sites, whether to extend, refurbish or build new and the key **Project Outcomes** as well as initial considerations for the **Project Programme** and assembling the project team.

### Sustainability Aspirations

The client's aspirations for sustainability, which may include additional objectives, measures or specific levels of performance in relation to international standards, as well as details of specific demands in relation to operational or facilities management issues.

The **Sustainability Strategy** will be prepared in response to the **Sustainability Aspirations** and will include specific additional items, such as an energy plan and ecology plan and the design life of the building, as appropriate.

### Sustainability Strategy

The strategy for delivering the **Sustainability Aspirations**.

### Technology Strategy

The strategy established at the outset of a project that sets out technologies, including Building Information Modelling (BIM) and any supporting processes, and the specific software packages that each member of the project team will use. Any interoperability issues can then be addressed before the design phases commence.

This strategy also considers how information is to be communicated (by email, file transfer protocol (FTP) site or using a managed third party common data environment) as well as the file formats in which information will be provided. The **Project Execution Plan** records agreements made.

### Work in Progress

**Work in Progress** is ongoing design work that is issued between designers to facilitate the iterative coordination of each designer's output. Work issued as **Work in Progress** is signed off by the internal design processes of each designer and is checked and coordinated by the lead designer.

# Index